HEALTHY PLACES,
HEALTHY PEOPLE

A Handbook for Culturally Competent Community Nursing Practice

Books Published by the Honor Society of Nursing, Sigma Theta Tau International

The Nurse's Etiquette Advantage: How Professional Etiquette Can Advance Your Nursing Career, Pagana, 2008.

Johns Hopkins Nursing Evidence-Based Practice Model and Guidelines, Newhouse, Dearholt, Poe, Pugh, and White, 2007.

Nursing Without Borders: Values, Wisdom, Success Markers, Weinstein and Brooks, 2007.

Synergy: The Unique Relationship Between Nurses and Patients, Curley, 2007.

Conversations With Leaders: Frank Talk From Nurses (and Others) on the Front Lines of Leadership, Hansen-Turton, Sherman, and Ferguson, 2007.

Pivotal Moments in Nursing: Leaders Who Changed the Path of a Profession, Houser and Player, 2004 (Volume I) and 2007 (Volume II).

Shared Legacy, Shared Vision: The W.K. Kellogg Foundation and the Nursing Profession, Lynaugh, Smith, Grace, Sena, de Villalobos, and Hlalele, 2007.

Daily Miracles: Stories and Practices of Humanity and Excellence in Health Care, Briskin and Boller, 2006.

A Daybook for Nurse Leaders and Mentors, Sigma Theta Tau International, 2006.

When Parents Say No: Religious and Cultural Influences on Pediatric Healthcare Treatment, Linnard-Palmer, 2006.

Healthy Places, Healthy People: A Handbook for Culturally Competent Community Nursing Practice, Dreher, Shapiro, and Asselin, 2006.

The HeART of Nursing: Expressions of Creative Art in Nursing, Second Edition, Wendler, 2005.

Reflecting on 30 Years of Nursing Leadership: 1975-2005, Donley, 2005.

Technological Competency as Caring in Nursing, Locsin, 2005.

Making a Difference: Stories from the Point of Care, Volume 1, Hudacek, 2005.

A Daybook for Nurses: Making a Difference Each Day, Hudacek, 2004.

Making a Difference: Stories from the Point of Care, Volume 2, Hudacek, 2004.

Building and Managing a Career in Nursing: Strategies for Advancing Your Career, Miller, 2003.

Collaboration for the Promotion of Nursing, Briggs, Merk, and Mitchell, 2003.

Ordinary People, Extraordinary Lives: The Stories of Nurses, Smeltzer and Vlasses, 2003.

Stories of Family Caregiving: Reconsideration of Theory, Literature, and Life, Poirier and Ayres, 2002.

As We See Ourselves: Jewish Women in Nursing, Benson, 2001.

Cadet Nurse Stories: The Call for and Response of Women During World War II, Perry and Robinson, 2001.

Creating Responsive Solutions to Healthcare Change, McCullough, 2001.

The Language of Nursing Theory and Metatheory, King and Fawcett, 1997.

For more information and to order these books from the Honor Society of Nursing, Sigma Theta Tau International, visit the honor society's Web site at www.nursingsociety.org/publications, or go to www.nursingknowledge.org/stti/books, the Web site of Nursing Knowledge International, the honor society's sales and distribution division. Or, call 1.888.NKI.4.YOU (U.S. and Canada) or +1.317.634.8171 (Outside U.S. and Canada).

HEALTHY PLACES, HEALTHY PEOPLE

A Handbook for Culturally Competent Community Nursing Practice

Melanie Dreher, PhD, RN, FAAN, Dolores Shapiro, PhD, RN, and
Micheline Asselin, MPA, MSN, RN, CHPN

Sigma Theta Tau International
Honor Society of Nursing®

Sigma Theta Tau International

Editor-in-Chief: Jeff Burnham
Acquisitions Editor: Fay L. Bower, DNSc, RN, FAAN
Editors: Carla Hall, Jane Palmer
Proofreader: Linda Canter
Indexer: Angela Bess, RN
Designer: Rebecca Harmon
Typesetter: Rebecca Harmon

Printed in the United States of America
Printing and Binding by: Printing Partners

Sigma Theta Tau International
550 West North Street
Indianapolis, IN 46202 USA

Visit our Web site at **www.nursingknowledge.org/STTI/books** for more information on our books.

ISBN: 1-930538-17-0

Library of Congress Cataloging-in-Publication Data

Dreher, Melanie Creagan.
  Healthy places, healthy people : a cultural handbook for community nursing practice / Melanie Dreher, Dolores Shapiro, Micheline Asselin.
      p. ; cm.
  Includes bibliographical references and index.
  ISBN-13: 978-1-930538-17-7 (alk. paper)
  ISBN-10: 1-930538-17-0 (alk. paper)
 1. Community health nursing. 2. Community health services.
  [DNLM: 1. Community Health Nursing. 2. Community Health Services. WY 106 D771h 2005] I. Shapiro, Dolores. II. Asselin, Micheline. III. Sigma Theta Tau International. IV. Title.

RT98.D74 2005
610.73'43--dc22

                                                                        2005026732

Second printing
2008

DEDICATION

This book is dedicated to my dear friend, Dr. Jagna Wojcicka Sharff, whose life and career were devoted to understanding people in communities and how they live and work and grow and love. Her work as an anthropologist inspired my work as a nurse. Affectionately known as "the people's Jagna," she touched the lives of millions and made them better (including mine).

—Melanie Dreher, PhD, RN, FAAN

ACKNOWLEDGEMENTS

We are deeply indebted to the communities in which we worked and the residents and institutions that opened their doors and hearts to our students. The University of Massachusetts students, themselves, who embraced a new way to nurse and enthusiastically set about creating healthier places for people to have healthier lives, also deserve our gratitude.

The genesis of this book can be traced to our professors: Dr. Conrad Arensberg, whose concepts of community and culture are foundational to our treatise; Dr. Lambros Comitas, whose teachings about the sociocultural complexity of local life framed our interventions; and Dr. Ralph Holloway, whose clarification of current concepts relative to the issue of race is preliminary to our discourse on social justice and health disparities. We are grateful for their wisdom.

There are not sufficient ways to thank Wendy Mains, Maureen Groden, Ken Culp, and Sue Licher for their careful reading and thoughtful comments on the manuscript. And finally, we are very grateful to our families and colleagues, and to each other, for unrelenting patience and support.

Melanie Creagan Dreher, PhD, RN, FAAN
Dolores J. Shapiro, PhD, RN
Micheline Asselin, MPA, MSN, RN, CHPN

About the Authors

Melanie Dreher, PhD, RN, FAAN

Melanie Dreher is currently the John and Helen Kellogg Dean and professor at Rush University College of Nursing. An educator for more than 30 years, Dr. Dreher has championed nursing as the profession with the greatest potential to improve the health and well-being of people in communities. She has taught community assessment, analysis, and intervention at Columbia University, University of Miami, University of Massachusetts, and the University of Iowa. After graduating from Long Island College Hospital, she earned her bachelor's degree in nursing at Long Island University and her doctorate in anthropology at Columbia University and Teachers' College. Professor Dreher's extensive ethnographic research in the Caribbean has focused on communities as powerful determinants of the health and welfare of children and adults. She has represented nursing on hospital boards, citizen boards, and health insurance companies. Her community development work in Jamaica merited a citation from the United States ambassador. She held a visiting professorship at the University of West Indies. Dr. Dreher has published extensively on culture as an organizing concept in nursing education and practice.

Dolores Shapiro, PhD, RN

Dolores Shapiro is a nurse and anthropologist who has taught graduate and undergraduate nursing students at the University of Nevada at Reno, Columbia University, University of Massachusetts at Amherst, and Rutgers University. She received her bachelor of science in nursing from the State University of New York at Plattsburgh, her master's degree in psychosocial nursing from the University of Washington, and her doctoral degree in cultural anthropology from Columbia University. Pursuing her interest in medical anthropology and the anthropology of religion, she has focused her research on spirit possession, race relations, and drug consumption. Dr. Shapiro has conducted community-based ethnographic research in New York City, Jamaica, and northeastern Brazil. Her practice includes school health, mental health, occupational health, and community program development in such diverse places as New York, Germany, Hawaii, Oregon, New Mexico, and Massachusetts. She also is a volunteer with the National Nurse Response Team of the Federal Emergency Management Agency. She currently resides and works in New York City.

MICHELINE ASSELIN, MPA, MSN, RN, CHPN

Micheline Asselin currently teaches community health nursing at the University of Massachusetts at Amherst to RNs completing their bachelor's degree. She has worked as a practitioner, teacher, and administrator in community health and hospice nursing for 40 years and now serves in an advisory capacity to several community and public health agencies. Throughout her career, Professor Asselin has mobilized students to become community activists to build the capacity of communities to promote healthy populations. As director of the home care program for the first American hospice, she lobbied effectively for federal reimbursement of hospice care. Professor Asselin is a graduate of the Springfield Hospital School of Nursing. She earned a bachelor's degree at the University of Massachusetts at Amherst, and a master's degree in public administration and a master's in nursing from the University of Hartford in Connecticut.

TABLE OF CONTENTS

INTRODUCTION XIV

PART I: COMMUNITY HEALTH PRACTICE: ITS FEATURES AND FOUNDATIONS 1
    References 2

CHAPTER 1: THE CULTURAL FRAMEWORK OF COMMUNITY HEALTH 3
    Cultural Competence in Nursing Practice 5
    Conservatism in Community Nursing 8
    The Scientific Basis of Community Health Nursing 10
    Summary 14
    References 15

CHAPTER 2: THE CULTURAL FOUNDATION OF COMMUNITY HEALTH 19
    What Is Community Health Nursing? 20
    What Is a Healthy Community? 20
    What Is a Community? 22
    Population 23
    Environment 24
    Culture 24
    Who Is the Client in Community Health Nursing? 25
    Populations 25
    Communities 27
    Building Community Capacity Through Cultural Knowledge 28
    Community Nursing Practice 29
    Assessment and Analysis 30
    Community Planning and Intervention 31
    Evaluation 33
    The Nurse-Client Relationship 33
    Community Nursing Values and Conflicts 35
    Community Health Nursing: A Work in Progress 37
    References 45

PART II: CULTURE AND HEALTH ASSESSMENT FOR COMMUNITY HEALTH
    PRACTICE   49
    References 50

CHAPTER 3: COMMUNITY CULTURAL ASSESSMENT 51
   Community Cultural Assessment Process 54
      Gathering Community Data 54
   The Community as a Place in Time 61
      Spatial Dimensions of Community Life 62
      Size and Boundaries 62
      Regional Position 63
      Geophysical and Climate Factors 65
      Land Use 66
      Housing 68
      Transportation and Communication 69
      Mental Maps 71
      Community History 73
      Cyclical Population Movement 74
      Economic Cycle 75
      Psychological Cycles 76
      Cyclical Crises 78
   The Community as a Population 80
      Temporary Subpopulations 82
      Biological Composition: Age and Sex 82
      Racial and Ethnic Groups 84
      Occupation, Income, and Education Level 87
      Residential and Household Characteristics 89
      Managing Population Data 90
   The Community as a Social System 91
      Economic Institutions 93
      Government, Politics, and Law Enforcement 94
      Domestic Organization 97
      Religious Institutions 100
      Educational Institutions 102
      Recreation 104
      Voluntary Organizations 106
      Horizontal Stratification 108
      Vertical Segmentation 110
   Managing Social System Data 112
   Summary 112
      References 113

CHAPTER 4: COMMUNITY HEALTH ASSESSMENT 119
  What Is a Healthy Community? 120
  Measuring the Health of Communities. 120
  Analyzing the Health of Communities 124
  Assessing the Health of Populations. 124
  Biostatistical Measures of Population Health 125
    Mortality Rates. 127
    Morbidity Rates 128
  Epidemiological Studies of Population Health 130
  Community Health Status: Vulnerable Groups. 134
    Infectious Diseases 135
    Chronic Diseases 136
    Chronic Disability 137
    Behavioral Health 138
    Maternal-Child Health 139
    Maternal-Child Health Behavior 140
    School-Age Child Health 142
    Worker Health 143
    Unhealthy Behaviors 145
  Population Health Status Indicators 146
  Health-Related Data. 151
  Assessing the Health of the Environment 154
    Air Pollution 156
    Water Pollution 158
    Food Contamination 160
    Waste Management 161
    Solid Waste. 161
    Sewage 163
    Radioactive Waste 164
    Chemical Waste 166
    Noise Pollution 168
    Disease Vectors. 169
    Disasters. 170
    Crime. 172
    Accidents 174
    Housing Construction 175

Community Buildings. *176*
Energy Management. *178*
Overview 179
Assessing the Infrastructure for Prevention and Health Promotion 180
Public Health Institutions. *182*
Health Departments. *184*
Personal Health Services and Public Health 186
Healthy Planning Agencies. *187*
Healthcare Financing *187*
Beliefs About Public Health *188*
Alternative Health Systems. *190*
Summary 191
References *192*

PART III: ACTION AND ADVOCACY IN COMMUNITY HEALTH PRACTICE 197
References *198*

CHAPTER 5: CULTURE-BASED PLANNING FOR COMMUNITY HEALTH 199
The Value of Community Health Planning. 200
Trends in Health Planning 201
Resource-Based Planning 202
Population-Based Planning. 205
Culture-Based Planning 207
Community Participation in Health Planning. 210
Creating a Culture-Based Community Health Plan 213
Goals *214*
Priorities. *216*
Measurable Outcomes *218*
Operational Plans *219*
Cost-Effectiveness. *220*
Evaluation *221*
Culture, Change, and Planning. 222
References *223*

CHAPTER 6: COMMUNITY PRACTICE IMPLEMENTATION:
  CULTURE-BASED LEADERSHIP............................225
 Implementation, Leadership, and Community Nursing Practice........... 226
 Implementation Strategies...................................... 226
 The Complexity of Community Clients 229
 Creating Community Relations: Constituencies and Coalitions 233
 Implementing the Healthy Community Agenda 238
 The Case Statement: Formulating the Culturally Effective Message 246
 Summary 248
 References *250*

EPILOGUE...253
 References *255*

INDEX 257

INTRODUCTION

This is a book about community health practice. It is intended to help nursing students use the concept of culture to understand how communities work. In many ways, it is a "how-to" book—a practical guide for all nurses learning to care for the health of whole communities. We assert that healthy places (both social and physical) are fundamental to healthy people. The goal of community nursing practice is to build the capacity of communities to protect the health and welfare of its citizens so they can reduce or eliminate their reliance on health (or really *illness)* care.

> **The goal of community nursing is to enhance community capacity for assuring a robust physical and social environment that will promote health and prevent illness.**

This does not mean we challenge the role of the nurse as a direct care provider either in the home or in other noninstitutional settings. Nor does it mean nursing should abdicate its social responsibility to care for the sick. It does mean, however, that community health nursing is the specialized area of practice entrusted with the *health* of the entire *public*—not just those who are sick and not just those who have insurance or can afford to pay. It means the goal of community nursing is to *enhance community capacity* for assuring a robust physical and social environment that will promote health and prevent illness.

In this book, we argue that community health nursing is defined by orientation rather than by setting. For example, a nurse working in the oncology service of a tertiary care setting who mobilizes health policy for cancer prevention, supports community education for early identification of cancer, establishes self-help programs for cancer survivors, and links the families of cancer patients to community services has a strong community orientation. In contrast, nurses whose practice in a prenatal clinic is limited to assessing and counseling expectant mothers, without any interest in policies regarding ethnic disparities in low birth weight or programs that provide parenting skills, day-care programs, or family planning services are not community health-oriented, even though they work in community-based settings. In fact, while much is made of hospital versus community, the distinction between them is not a factor that defines community practice. The hospital is simply another community institution (not unlike churches, schools, factories, etc.), and the patients in them also are community residents. Our goal is to offer a perspective that prepares some students for careers in community health nursing and assists all students to expand the scope of their practices and acquire a more comprehensive understanding of their role in society, wherever they work.

Although nursing takes nourishment from many disciplines, the two that have most informed this text are anthropology and epidemiology. In addition to being nurses, two of the authors of this text are anthropologists, and the third has a degree in healthcare policy. Therefore, it is not surprising that a sociocultural paradigm prevails throughout the text, with emphasis on the collection and application of "local" knowledge, a quest for cultural sensitivity, and a community-oriented practice.

This text places nurses at the center of the health team, solving problems and monitoring, designing, planning, and directing the care of whole populations. It speaks to the responsibility of nurses to shape the future of healthcare. Some may regard this as an idealistic approach to public or community health nursing and argue there are few places in which we practice in the manner recommended here. We regard this as an asset rather than a shortcoming. Educators have an obligation to teach their students not only what is, but also what can and should be. We have a responsibility not only to assist nursing graduates to take positions in the existing healthcare system, but also to have the vision and ability to forge new roles, negotiate more effective healthcare systems, and ultimately to create healthier communities. The fact that there are few places in which true community health nursing is being practiced should not discourage us; it should energize us. The companion covenant, of course, is to provide students with the practical concepts and skills needed to reconstruct healthcare systems and promote global health. Thus, while we are unabashedly idealistic about our goals, we have tried to be painstakingly realistic about our strategies for achieving them. Impractical tactics and failed results only serve to discourage nurses and eventually to make them stop trying.

In this book, we offer students a public-health improvement strategy that can be applied to any community at any time. It is about assessment, analysis, and action to build community capacity. Students will learn how to view and interpret community strength, as well as vulnerability, and to formulate and implement interventions. This culturally grounded community perspective permits nurses to anticipate and plan for a healthy future. It is one large exercise in critical thinking.

Engaging in a practice that has the potential to improve the health of individuals, families, whole communities, and even nations for generations to come is a momentous undertaking. It is certainly as challenging, demanding, and exciting as working in an intensive care unit, an emergency room, or in labor and delivery. We hope this book conveys the personal gratification and fulfillment that can be derived from a career with almost limitless possibilities for fundamental and far-reaching social change.

Melanie Dreher, PhD, RN, FAAN
Dolores Shapiro, PhD, RN
Micheline Asselin, MPA, MSN, RN, CHPN

FEATURES

OBJECTIVES

Each chapter starts out with objectives, giving the student and instructor a way to measure progress and to reinforce the critical-thinking skills offered within each chapter.

ASSESSMENT INSTRUMENT

The assessment instrument presented in the boxes throughout chapters 3 and 4 is a great resource for the student, instructor, and practitioner.

CHAPTER-LEVEL CONTENT

CHAPTER 1—"THE CULTURAL FRAMEWORK OF COMMUNITY HEALTH"

This chapter frames the concept of community health nursing by providing a solid understanding of culture and an exploration of the scientific foundations of community health nursing.

Chapter 1 Objectives

- Describe the significance of culture as an organizing concept in community nursing.

- Compare anthropology and epidemiology with regard to their units of analysis.

- Specify the advantages of a community approach to nursing practice.

- Explain the ecological fallacy intrinsic to commonly held notions of cultural competence and how it may actually impede care.

CHAPTER 2—"THE CULTURAL FOUNDATION OF COMMUNITY HEALTH"

This chapter provides concepts and assumptions that guide and distinguish community health nursing practice. It explores population, community, and health in conceptual terms.

Chapter 2 Objectives

- Identify the goals and unique features of community health nursing.

- Explain how health, community, population, and culture work together as guiding concepts in community health nursing.

- Describe the assumptions on which protecting and maintaining the health of communities are founded.

- Specify the advantages of a community approach to nursing practice.

- Depict the value orientation of community health and its relation to nursing practice and education.

- Trace the emergence of community nursing practice.

CHAPTER 3—"COMMUNITY CULTURAL ASSESSMENT"

This chapter provides the student with the knowledge and tools to conduct a community cultural assessment.

Chapter 3 Objectives

- Identify the sources and methods of data gathering about the cultural capital of a community.

- Describe the spatial and temporal dimensions of community life that impact on health and health services.

- Delineate the sociodemographic characteristics of populations that are significant for determining community health status.

- Identify the major components of social organization that impact on health and healthcare.

- Apply the methods for analyzing cultural assessment data for formulating a healthy community agenda.

CHAPTER 4—"COMMUNITY HEALTH ASSESSMENT"

This chapter provides the student with the knowledge and tools to conduct a community health assessment.

Chapter 4 Objectives

- Identify sources of population health assessment data.

- Interpret health data using biostatistician and epidemiological measures.

- Determine the health status of a population.

- Examine the health of the environment.

- Identify the cultural capital dedicated to the pursuit of health.

- Compare the community's health institutions in terms of primary, secondary, and tertiary prevention.

CHAPTER 5—"CULTURE-BASED PLANNING FOR COMMUNITY HEALTH"

This chapter describes the basic principles and strategies for using assessment data to identify a health problem and develop a culturally appropriate plan for its solution.

Chapter 5 Objectives

- Identify the value of health planning.

- Compare culture-based planning with resource-based and population-based planning.

- Outline the process of culture-based planning.

- Distinguish between an activity plan and a strategic plan.

- Trace historical and current trends in health planning.

CHAPTER 6—"COMMUNITY PRACTICE IMPLEMENTATION: CULTURE-BASED LEADERSHIP"

This chapter continues with the analysis and utilization of assessment data for the purposes of community-specific action.

Chapter 6 Objectives

- Distinguish between the *conflict* and *consensus* models of public health action.

- Identify the special challenges of working with the community as client and the skills and theories needed.

- Describe the process of building a constituency.

- Describe the process of building a coalition.

- Distinguish between primary and secondary target groups in mobilizing community action.

- Prepare an effective public health message.

INSTRUCTORS

A teaching guide in PDF format is available free of charge to instructors who use this book in their classrooms. Contact us at customerservice@nursingknowledge.org to learn more or request your complimentary copy of the guide.

COMMUNITY HEALTH PRACTICE: ITS FEATURES AND FOUNDATIONS

Healthy communities are fundamental to healthy populations and the object of community practice intervention. But when confronted with the magnitude and complexity of the community-client, community health nurses often retreat to the interventions with which they are most familiar—specifically, personal health services. Thus in spite of more than two decades of critique (Butterfield, 1990; Dreher, 1982; Drevdahl, 1995; Kang, 1995), community health nursing continues to locate advocacy at the individual and family level. In their historical reluctance to move beyond personal health services, community health nurses have become "community assessors but personal intervenors, creating a paradox in which improving a community's health is accomplished through action aimed at individual behaviors rather than at the larger social and political vehicles" (Drevdahl, p. 13).

Flu immunizations, family planning clinics, nutritional counseling, smoking cessation, and prostate cancer screening are important and necessary public health activities. They are not sufficient, however, to build community capacity, i.e., a thriving, productive citizenry, residing in a healthy social and physical environment; nor are they sufficient to meet the two primary goals of *Healthy People 2010*—to eliminate health disparities and extend the quality and years of healthy life (U.S. Department of Health and Human Services, 2001). To accomplish the broad, far-reaching changes that will build sustainable, healthy places and populations, community advocacy must include large-scale social action (Atwood, Colditz, & Kawachi, 1997; Milio, 1975).

It is usually the case that the thorniest public health problems are those most deeply embedded in the traditions and structures of a community's culture. The growing epidemic of obese and overweight people, for example, is amazingly resistant to standard interventions. So in spite of public education, recreational facilities, nutritional disclosure on packaged food, and peer-support programs, not to mention any number of diets, behavior modification programs, hypnosis, and surgical interventions, the rate of obesity continues to grow, creating a national public health problem that has effectively reduced the quality and years of healthy life.

For most public health problems, there is no shortage of plans and projects. The debates over fluoridation, speed limits, cigarette advertisements, immunization, family planning, and gun control all demonstrate the significance of culture-bound values in shaping public health policy. The dilemmas encountered in advocating for healthy communities are attributable not to the lack of solutions, but rather to the difficulty in implementing those solutions within a complex community culture. Chapters 1 and 2 will explore and explain the fundamental concepts of culture, community, and population necessary to guide and frame community health practice.

REFERENCES

Atwood, K., Colditz, G.A., & Kawachi, I. (1997). From public health science to prevention policy. Placing science in its social and political contexts. *American Journal of Public Health, 87*(10), 1603-1606.

Butterfield, P.G. (1990). Thinking upstream: Nurturing a conceptual understanding of the societal context of health behavior. *Advances in Nursing Science, 12*(2), 1-8.

Dreher, M. (1982). The conflict of conservatism in public health nursing education. *Nursing Outlook, 30*(9), 504-509.

Drevdahl, D. (1995). Coming to voice: The power of emancipatory community interventions. *Advances in Nursing Science, 18*(2), 13-24.

Kang, R. (1995). Building community capacity for health promotion: A challenge for public health nurses. *Public Health Nursing, 12*(5), 312-318.

Milio, N. (1975). *The care of health in communities.* New York: Macmillan.

U.S. Department of Health and Human Services. (2001). *Healthy people 2010.* McLean, VA: International Medical Publishing.

THE CULTURAL FRAMEWORK OF COMMUNITY HEALTH

Community health nurses promote and protect the health of whole communities. Guided by the premise that a clean, safe, and supportive community will enhance the health of its individual citizens, community nursing is less about personal health services and more about building the community's capacity for a healthy and sustainable future.

CHAPTER 1 OBJECTIVES

- Describe the significance of culture as an organizing concept in community nursing.

- Compare anthropology and epidemiology with regard to their units of analysis.

- Specify the advantages of a community approach to nursing practice.

- Explain the ecological fallacy intrinsic to commonly held notions of cultural competence and how it may actually impede care.

Cultures are fluid and constantly changing vis-à-vis new environments and inconstant physical, social, economic, and political circumstances. Real cultural competence requires rejecting simplistic views of culture as monolithic and unchanging or that people are "frozen" in cultural traditions, unable to modify their behavior and learn new ways.

Culture is not a new concept in public health. The importance of knowing the community's culture to determine patterns of illness, health, and use of health services was documented almost 50 years ago in a landmark collection entitled *Health, Culture, and Community: Case Studies of Public Reactions to Health Programs* (Paul, 1955).

> If you wish to help a community improve its health, you must learn to think like the people. … To assume new health habits, it is wise to ascertain the existing habits, how these habits are linked to one another, what functions they perform, and what they mean to those who practice them. (p. 1)

Nor is culture new for public health nurses. In 1954, George Rosen advised:

> First and foremost comes a knowledge of the community and its people. This knowledge must be acquired and is just as important for successful public health work as is a knowledge of epidemiology or medicine. … The community health nurse … should be consciously aware of the way of life of the people, their goals in life, the motivations that make them do the things they do, the things in life that mean much or little to them. (p. 15)

Culture may be, in fact, the factor that most distinguishes nursing from medicine and other health professions (Dreher, 1996; Leininger, 1989). For decades, nursing has been defined as the diagnosis and treatment of human *responses* to health and illness (American Nurses Association, 1980), which obliges nurses to include culture among their guiding concepts. Individuals vary in their responses to disease and also to birth, death, infirmity, developmental transitions, treatment, and hospitalization; much of this variation can be traced to differences in the social and cultural contexts in which people live.

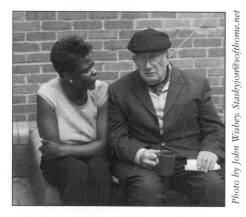

Photo by John Wisbey. Stashyjon@softhome.net

Unlike physicians—for whom a streptococcal infection is treated in the same manner whether the client is in Bangkok or London, or for whom hip replacement surgery is the same procedure in Kenya as in Canada—nurses must anticipate and accommodate the inevitable variation in clients' responses to an infection or to post-surgical recovery. Nurses understand that manifestations, acknowledgement, and management of even the most physiological responses are firmly embedded in the contexts of home and community, where clients and their families live their daily lives. Nursing is a cultural phenomenon;

most expressions of care and comfort are learned responses, derived in cultural context, and are subject to variation across ethnic and national groups.

When caring for individuals and families, nurses must find out more about their clients than just their disease, age, and sex. To be most therapeutic, nurses should know about their clients' ways of life, values, education, occupation, social status, family responsibilities, and the meanings these clients have given to their illness. Because of their holistic orientation, nurses are likely to have the most complete and in-depth knowledge of clients.

Likewise, with client-communities, community health nurses will want to know something more than the rate of HIV infection, the prevalence of diabetes, or the incidence of low birth-weight babies. They will also want to know about the community's economy, religious institutions, educational resources, commonly held values, social norms, power structures, justice systems, and the prevailing knowledge and beliefs about health and healthcare. In other words, they must understand the culture of the population to be served. Attention to culture can expose the determinants of health and illness, as well as identify community resources—or the *cultural capital*—that can be used to build the community's capacity for public health.

> As the United States continues to evolve as a multiethnic, culturally diverse society, a standard of cultural competence in all human services is wholesome, desirable, and consistent with principles of social justice.

CULTURAL COMPETENCE IN NURSING PRACTICE

In recent years, culturally competent care has emerged as the mantra of contemporary nursing practice (Campinha-Bacote & Munoz, 2001; Fahrenwald, Boysen, Fischer, & Maurer, 2001; Garity, 2000; Holland & Courtney, 1998; Leininger, 1989, 1997). Journals and books abound with formulas and instructions for students, educators, and clinicians on how to "become more culturally sensitive" and "celebrate diversity," preparing nurses for a practice world in which ethnic and racial diversity is the norm. Acknowledging the dramatic changes in ethnic composition that challenge a healthcare system is long overdue. As the United States continues to evolve as a multiethnic, culturally diverse society, a standard of cultural competence in all human services is wholesome, desirable, and consistent with principles of social justice. On the other hand, cultural competence is not well understood and is subject to many interpretations. Culturally competent care, as an outcome, is difficult to measure as well as to teach. Moreover, culture has become a term used to describe almost any kind of group beliefs or behavior. Given the complexity of culture and its importance for nursing, it is useful to critically examine the notion of cultural competence and what it means for community nursing.

Until fairly recently, health professionals have tended to identify culture as something that occurs in other societies or in so-called ethnic communities. But all communities, including those of health providers, have a culture. Perhaps even more problematic is the lack of understanding of the distinction between ethnicity as an individual characteristic and culture as a group characteristic. The term *culture* refers to the learned patterns of behavior and range of beliefs attributed to a specific group that are passed on through generations. It includes ways of life, norms and values, social institutions, and a shared construction of the physical world. While cultural groups are composed of individuals, most members go through life assuming only some features of their identified culture. Some may embrace cultural norms, while others may reject them; still others may apply them situationally. Thus individuals with the same ethnic background may exhibit varying levels of adherence to traditional cultural norms.

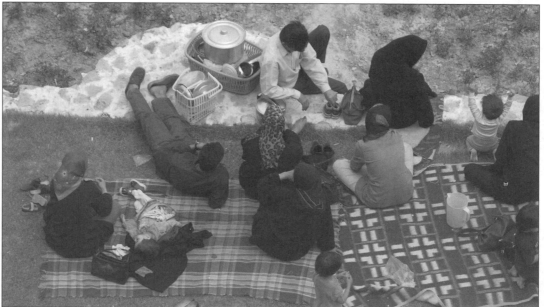

Photo by Mira Pavlakovic, Ozalj, Croatia.

It is generally understood that culture, in its most comprehensive meaning, pertains to groups. The problem is that healthcare typically is dispensed to individuals. When information about groups (cultures) is used to make predictions about individuals (clients), it is termed an *ecological fallacy* (Bernard, 2002; Dreher & MacNaughton, 2002). Ironically, in an attempt to be culturally sensitive, nurses and physicians often act on information that simply may not apply to specific individuals and could compromise clinical effectiveness. If, for example, the normative definition of female physical beauty in a particular culture is 5 feet tall and 180 pounds, it would be easy to dismiss obesity in women as simply a cultural phenomenon and ignore the possibility of physiological or psychological pathology. While cultural norms regarding desired female body mass may help explain the presence of obesity in a particular group, they cannot be presumed to account for obesity in a particular woman. The nurse still would not really know whether, and to what extent, obesity in a particular woman was attributable to cultural, physiological, or psychological factors, or a combination of all these factors.

In addition to a narrow conception of culture, making assumptions about cultural uniformity often fails to account for the shifting nature of a culture. Although cultures differ in the speed with which change occurs and the degree of internal variation, few could be described as static and/or homogenous. Cultures are fluid and constantly changing vis-à-vis new environments and inconstant physical, social, economic, and political circumstances. Real cultural competence requires rejecting simplistic views of culture as monolithic and unchanging or that people are "frozen" in cultural traditions, unable to modify their behavior and learn new ways.

> Ironically, in an attempt to be culturally sensitive, nurses and physicians often act on information that simply may not apply to specific individuals and could compromise clinical effectiveness.

While culture must be used judiciously in clinical practice, it is a potent and far-reaching concept in public health, where communities (groups) rather than individuals are the standard unit of intervention (Boyle, Szymanski, & Szymanski, 1992; Fahrenwald et al., 2001; Hagey, 1988; May, Mendelson, & Ferketich, 1995). Continuing with the earlier example, information about the norms and beliefs regarding female beauty is likely to have practical value in designing community-based responses to the high rates of obesity-related illness in specific populations. It also would have theoretical value in explaining the cultural determinants of obesity. Cultural knowledge about social rules, norms, and patterns of behavior provides guidance for social marketing and public education programs, for community-based health promotion initiatives, and for organizing personal health services for specific populations.

For community health nurses, real cultural competence is the extent to which they are effective in building community capacity—for example, assisting communities to identify, enhance, and deploy their cultural capital. *Cultural capital* is the arsenal of institutions, leaders, customs, knowledge, and values that forms the context for action and can be used to promote healthy, invested communities (Hopkins & Mehanna, 2000). This is not a very complicated concept. If, for example, it was desirable to increase the amount of available blood for use in the event of an emergency, it would not be necessary to go through the telephone book to solicit donors and convince each of them of their civic responsibilities. Rather, one would mobilize the leadership of local clubs and other voluntary organizations, provide them with the necessary literature and materials, and let those leaders convince their groups to donate blood as a worthy cause. The most successful public health initiatives and examples of real cultural competence are community-based programs that are targeted to specific social groups, engage community leaders, work through local institutions, and use culturally established channels of communication (Tripp-Reimer, 1999; Tripp-Reimer, Choi, Skemp-Kelly, & Enslein, 2001; U.S. Department of Health and Human Services [USDHHS], 2001a).

> For community health nurses, real cultural competence is the extent to which they are effective in building community capacity—for example, assisting communities to identify, enhance, and deploy their cultural capital.

CONSERVATISM IN COMMUNITY NURSING

It is not surprising nursing's interest in culture emerged in the public health arena. Tracing the development of culture as an organizing concept in nursing, Tripp-Reimer and Fox (1990) observed that interest in culture first appeared at the turn of the century among public health nurses who reported differences in life and health patterns between existing communities and immigrant communities. Later, when nursing education was moved from hospitals to universities, an increased exposure to social sciences, such as anthropology, permitted nurses to acquire a broader understanding of the determinants of health and illness. Those determinants include social and economic dislocations that keep some communities on uneven footing, creating inequalities and group disparities in health status.

Unfortunately, instead of using cultural knowledge to generate the "culturally transformative" (Tripp-Reimer et al., 2001), far-reaching reform that could ameliorate some of the major health problems of society, nurses have focused on the prevention of disease almost exclusively through the encouragement of individuals to adopt healthy lifestyle behaviors. Rather than working at the policy level to change the political and economic institutions that permit the conditions of poor public health to exist, community nurses have tended to advocate for individual clients and their families, while neglecting the system-level action needed to promote sustainable and healthy communities. Nurses have helped communities adjust to inadequate housing, unsatisfactory waste disposal, and dangerous traffic patterns but have neglected the system-level action needed to truly improve the health of the public. Even if nurses are committed to addressing health disparities by rendering culturally competent care to individual patients and their families (SmithBattle, Diekemper, & Drake, 1999), their best intentions are no match for the power structure that perpetuates inequalities in health and access.

Chafey (1996) addresses this problem in a critique of "caring" in its application to public health:

> Nurses must care about what happens to groups of citizens, as well as particular clients. ... Although proponents of "caring" seem to have drawn a distinction between an ethic of justice and an ethic of care, this is bipolar, even antithetical. Building the health of communities requires universal application of the principles of justice. It further requires that nurses care enough about their communities and the individuals in them to do battle in political, social, and economic arenas. (p. 15)

Many argue the political conservatism that has characterized nursing—even community nursing—is attributable to the socialization of nurses into passive roles and their lack of assertiveness. A more probable explanation, however, lies in the nursing profession's almost exclusive concentration on individuals and families as the unit of nursing care. Typically, nursing education emphasizes nurse-client and nurse-family relationships. Thus, there are many excellent clinicians who are not necessarily well prepared to manage the organization or context of care or to function in the public or political arena. With the exception of culture, which often is misapplied to the care of individuals, nursing education generally does not include theories that apply to group- or community-level behavior

> Without an arsenal of theories that recognizes whole communities as a fundamental unit of society, nurses are not equipped to take group-level action, resulting in a political conservatism that continues to characterize professional nursing.

(Tripp-Reimer, 1999). This is both a cause and a product of the traditional focus on individual care. Even in community nursing, theories grounded in psychology (e.g., anomie, symbolic interaction, cognitive dissonance, and health belief models) continue to dominate nursing education and practice along with the emphasis on personal health services.

Without an arsenal of theories that recognizes whole communities as a fundamental unit of public health, nurses are not equipped to take group-level action, and political conservatism continues to characterize professional nursing. Although formal definitions of community health nursing identify geopolitically based populations as the unit of service, students of community health nursing often never learn how to go beyond assessment to apply that concept in their practice (Butterfield, 1990; Dreher, 1982; Drevdahl, 1995).

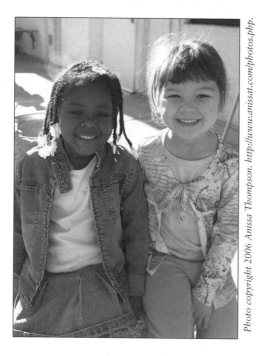

Photo copyright 2006 Anissa Thompson. http://www.anissat.com/photos.php.

A brilliant and timeless example of what nurses can do when they focus on creating healthy communities and not just on personal health services is presented in *9226 Kercheval Street* (Milio, 1970). While working as a young visiting nurse in an inner-city community in Detroit, MI, Milio discovered the most effective assistance she could provide to the mothers on public assistance was to help them be independent wage earners. To do this, she partnered with those mothers to establish a cooperative day-care center where they could safely leave their children while they entered the workforce. Fighting many policy and financial battles, Milio helped her clients to initiate a day-care center and run it independently. Most importantly, she engaged citizens in community-level action in which they identified and used existing community resources to create a healthier, more wholesome environment for children.

THE SCIENTIFIC BASIS OF COMMUNITY HEALTH NURSING

Traditionally, the fundamental science of public health has been epidemiology. Grounded in the notion that the individual is the basic unit of society, epidemiological research identifies variations among populations in the distribution of diseases and health problems to understand the etiology of diseases. The variables that are discovered to be associated with a particular disease are identified as risk factors, which then are used to guide public health intervention. A simple and well-known example is the identification of tobacco smoking as a risk factor for lung cancer. The goal of public health is to reduce the incidence and prevalence of lung cancer by reducing the incidence and prevalence of tobacco smoking. The contributions of epidemiology for improving the health of the public through identification of risk factors and disease prevention are profound and have done more to en-hance the health of the public in the last century than all of the efforts of clinical medicine.

With increasing acknowledgement of the influence of culture on health and illness, epidemiological studies have expanded the usual biological risk factors to include social and cultural determinants. In most instances, however, epidemiology has approached the concept of culture as an individual risk factor (ethnicity or national origin) to be correlated in large-scale studies with other risk factors (income, sex, genetic history, education) in the search for the cause of disease. Being African American, for example, is a risk factor for hypertension; being American Indian is a risk factor for diabetes. Such correlations, however, do not distinguish *ethnicity,* an *individual* trait or characteristic, from *culture,* a characteristic of *groups* that describes community-level patterns of beliefs, behaviors, and institutions. Taken out of context, these correlations do not explain how identified risk factors are articulated in the complex community cultures where people live out their daily lives. What is it, for example, that puts American Indians at greater risk for diabetes or African Americans at greater risk for hypertension? Knowing that tobacco smoking and lung cancer are highly correlated will not be sufficient to reduce the incidence and prevalence of lung cancer and other pulmonary diseases unless we also understand the cultural significance of smoking cigarettes, the number of people who earn a living growing tobacco and producing cigarettes, and the political strength of the tobacco industry.

With the development of medical anthropology as a discipline, there has been a mounting awareness that the relationship between health status and social status cannot be explained solely with reference to genetic variables, lifestyle choices, or differences in access to health services (Corin, 1994; Dressler, 1982, 1985). As the evidence accumulates, we have begun to have a better understanding that health inequalities are rooted in community culture, where the conditions of disparities are most evident. Unlike epidemiological studies, which use the individual, aggregated in populations, as the unit of analysis, medical anthropologists study whole communities as the context for understanding the way in which culture influences health and illness. There is, for example, increasing evidence that the health of individuals is directly linked to the capacity of the community to engage its citizens in a network of social relationships. A well-known study about mortality in

Alameda County, CA (Berkman & Syme, 1979), found the most significant predictor of mortality was how socially connected individuals were, independent of the usual risk factors such as smoking, diet, and exercise.

Similarly, a study of low infant birth weight in six Chicago neighborhoods showed neighborhood characteristics such as housing costs, crowding, community age distributions, and cultural homogeneity were more predictive of inequalities in maternal-infant health than individual risk factors such as race, ethnicity, and socioeconomic status. Surprisingly, neighborhoods with higher-cost housing had a higher rate of low infant birth weight than did neighborhoods with more crowded housing and a higher concentration of young African-American residents (Roberts, 1997). These findings were explained by better social support for pregnant women in the more crowded but culturally homogenous neighborhoods and by the availability of more disposable income (for food and care) in neighborhoods with lower-cost housing.

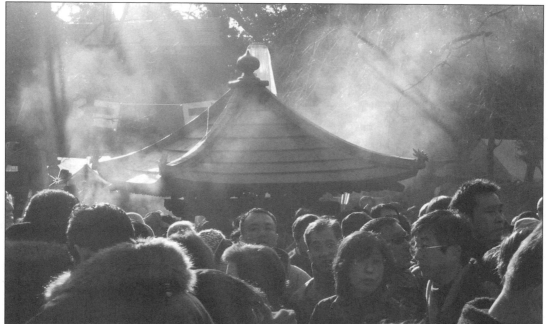

Photo by Aron Kremer, Japan.

In anthropology, the unit of analysis is the cultural group—frequently framed as community (Arensberg, 1961). Using ethnographic methods such as participant observation, kinship analysis, institutional analysis, and network analysis, anthropologists set about identifying the constellation of conditions and systems in communities that produce health and illness. Ethnographers approach culture not as an individual risk factor (ethnicity), but as "the matrix of collective influences that shape the lives of groups and individuals" (Corin, 1994, p. 101). Compared with the concrete reality of a population, culture is conceptual and therefore more difficult to study empirically than populations. Usually, culture is approached through in-depth studies in single communities that permit an identification of the linkages among the various aspects of local life that explain patterns of health and illness.

The importance of both populations and communities in providing a comprehensive and informed approach to growing and sustaining healthy communities has necessitated expanding the scientific orientation of public health practice to include anthropology as well as epidemiology. The determinants of health are multiple and complex and are embedded in the cultural context of communities in which individuals and families live. Yet we have relied almost exclusively on an epidemiological orientation in which populations have been used as the basic unit of analysis to identify not only the causes but also the solutions for poor community health (Cwikel, 1994). When ethnographic studies are deployed in conjunction with epidemiological studies, they provide a mutually reinforcing approach to understanding the causes of and solutions for poor health.

In this book, an anthropological approach is employed in which ethnographic methods, using communities as the units of analysis, are complemented by population-based epidemiological studies. Nurses, with their intimate and comprehensive knowledge of community life, are extraordinarily well positioned to be ethnographers—collecting, analyzing, and then acting on data that usually are difficult and expensive for public health officers and social scientists to flush out. Indeed, the description of the role of anthropologists in global health (Helman, 2001)—to ensure the cultural relevance of public health programs; identify community resources; monitor the impact of community interventions; mobilize expertise for health planning and implementation; influence policymakers; advocate for communities at state, national, and international levels; and continuously develop better, more efficient ways to assess communities—also describes the role of community health nurses.

> People do not live out their lives in populations. Nor do they live out their lives in cultures. Rather, people live and experience health and illness in communities where circumstances generate conflict, where people do not always follow the rules, and where cultural norms and institutions fluctuate according to the exigencies of daily life.

SUMMARY

Healthy People 2010 is the third in a series of U.S. national agendas for improving the health of the public. Although it has many objectives related to disease prevention and health promotion, the two primary goals of the program are to increase the quality and years of healthy life and eliminate health disparities. *Healthy People 2010* is a nationwide agenda. However, the importance of communities, in which the determinants of health and the solutions to health problems are embedded within the cultural context of villages, towns, and neighborhoods, is acknowledged within the document. People do not live out their lives in populations. Nor do they live out their lives in cultures. Rather, people live and experience health and illness in communities where circumstances generate conflict, where people do not always follow the rules, and where cultural norms and institutions fluctuate according to the exigencies of daily life. Communities constitute the matrix in which health and illness are produced and expressed, and where effective intervention occurs. It is here that nurses get things done, meet with individuals and groups, and use local institutions and cultural norms to create and accomplish a *Healthy People* agenda. *It is here where nurses identify and deploy the cultural capital required to build community capacity.* In the following chapters, it will be made clear that the concept of culture is fundamental to community health. Culture is what turns a population and a place into a community. While culture is not directly observable, it is the conceptual lens through which we come to understand the local community and its impact on health (USDHHS, 2001a, 2001b).

> Culture is what turns a population and a place into a community.

REFERENCES

American Nurses Association. (1980). *Nursing: A social policy statement.* Kansas City, MO: Author.

Arensberg, C. (1961). The community as object and sample. *American Anthropologist, 63,* 241-264.

Berkman, L.F., & Syme, L.S. (1979). Social networks, host resistance, and mortality: A nine-year follow-up study of Alameda County residents. *American Journal of Epidemiology, 109*(2), 186-204.

Bernard, H.R. (2002). *Research methods in anthropology: Qualitative and quantitative approaches* (3rd ed.). Walnut Creek, CA: Alta Mira Press.

Boyle, J.S., Szymanski, M.T., & Szymanski, M.E. (1992). Improving home health care for the Navajo. *Nursing Connections, 5*(4), 3-13.

Butterfield, P.G. (1990). Thinking upstream: Nurturing a conceptual understanding of the societal context of health behavior. *Advances in Nursing Science, 12*(2), 1-8.

Campinha-Bacote, J., & Munoz, C. (2001). A guiding framework for delivering culturally competent services in case management. *The Case Manager, 12*(2), 48-52.

Chafey, K. (1996). "Caring" is not enough: Ethical paradigms for community-based care. *Nursing and Health Care Perspectives on Community, 17*(1), 10-15.

Corin, E. (1994). The social and cultural matrix of health and disease. In R.G. Evans, M.L. Barer, & T.R. Marmor (Eds.), *Why are some people healthy and others not?: The determinants of health of populations* (pp. 93-132). New York: Aldine DeGruyter.

Cwikel, J.G. (1994). After epidemiological research: What next? Community action for health promotion. *Public Health Reviews, 22*(3-4), 375-394.

Dreher, M. (1982). The conflict of conservatism in public health nursing education. *Nursing Outlook, 30*(9), 504-509.

Dreher, M. (1996). Nursing: A cultural phenomenon. *Reflections on Nursing Leadership, 1*(4), 4.

Dreher, M., & MacNaughton, N. (2002). Cultural competence in nursing: Fallacy or foundation? *Nursing Outlook, 50*(5), 181-186.

Dressler, W.W. (1982). *Hypertension and culture change: Acculturation and disease in the West Indies.* New York: Redgrave.

Dressler, W.W. (1985). Psychosomatic symptoms, stress, and modernization: A model. *Culture, Medicine, and Psychiatry. 9*(3), 257-286.

Drevdahl, D. (1995). Coming to voice: The power of emancipatory community interventions. *Advances in Nursing Science, 18*(2), 13-24.

Fahrenwald, N., Boysen, R., Fischer, C., & Maurer, R. (2001). Developing cultural competence in the baccalaureate nursing student: A population-based project with the Hutterites. *Journal of Transcultural Nursing, 12*(1), 48-55.

Garity, J. (2000). Cultural competence in patient education. *Caring, 19*(3), 18-20.

Hagey, R. (1988). Retrospective on the culture concept. *Recent Advances in Nursing, 20,* 1-10.

Helman, C. (2001). *Culture, Health, and Illness.* London: Arnold.

Holland, L., & Courtney, R. (1998). Increasing cultural competence with the Latino community. *Journal of Community Health Nursing, 15*(1), 45-53.

Hopkins, N., & Mehanna, S.R. (2000). Social action against everyday pollution in Egypt. *Human Organization, 59*(2), 245-254.

Leininger, M. (1989). Leininger's theory of nursing: Cultural care diversity and universality. *Nursing Science Quarterly, 1*(4), 152-160.

Leininger, M. (1997). Transcultural nursing research to transform nursing education and practice. *Image: Journal of Nursing Scholarship, 29,* 341-347.

May, K.M., Mendelson, C., & Ferketich, S. (1995). Community empowerment in rural health care. *Public Health Nursing, 12*(1), 25-30.

Milio, N. (1970). *9226 Kercheval Street: The storefront that did not burn.* Ann Arbor, MI: University of Michigan Press.

Paul, B. (Ed.). (1955). *Health, culture, and community: Case studies of public reactions to health programs.* New York: Russell Sage Foundation.

Roberts, E. (1997). Neighborhood social environments and the distribution of low birth weight in Chicago. *American Journal of Public Health, 87*(4), 597-603.

Rosen, G. (1954). The community and the health officer: A working team. *American Journal of Public Health, 44*(1), 14-17.

SmithBattle, L., Diekemper, M., & Drake, M.A. (1999). Articulating the culture and tradition of community health nursing. *Public Health Nursing, 16*(3), 215-222.

Tripp-Reimer, T. (1999). Cultural interventions for ethnic groups of color. In A.S. Hinshaw, S. Feetham, & J. Shaver (Eds.), *Handbook of clinical nursing research* (pp. 107-123). Thousand Oaks, CA: Sage.

Tripp-Reimer, T., Choi, E., Skemp-Kelly, L., & Enslein, J. (2001). Cultural barriers to care: Inverting the problem. *Diabetes Spectrum, 14*(1), 13-22.

Tripp-Reimer, T., & Fox, S. (1990). Beyond the concept of culture. In J. McCloskey & H. Grace (Eds.), *Current Issues in Nursing* (pp. 542-547). London: Blackwell Scientific.

U.S. Department of Health and Human Services. (2001a). *Cultural competence works. Using cultural competence to improve the quality of health care for diverse populations and add value to managed care arrangements.* (Government publications 98-0372). Merrifield, VA: Author.

U.S. Department of Health and Human Services. (2001b). *Healthy people 2010.* McLean, VA: International Medical Publishing.

2

THE CULTURAL FOUNDATION OF COMMUNITY HEALTH

A community is not just the sum of its individual citizens.

This chapter introduces community nursing practice, exploring its major features and explaining its guiding concepts, values, and orientation. While the notion of having a whole community as a client may be daunting at first, a systematic approach is introduced for assessing communities, determining intervention strategies, and evaluating progress. It will require a different way of thinking and a different set of skills than typically are used in clinical practice.

CHAPTER 2 OBJECTIVES

- Identify the goals and unique features of community health nursing.

- Explain how health, community, population, and culture work together as guiding concepts in community health nursing.

- Describe the assumptions on which protecting and maintaining the health of communities are founded.

- Specify the advantages of a community approach to nursing practice.

- Depict the value orientation of community health and its relation to nursing practice and education.

- Trace the emergence of community nursing practice.

WHAT IS COMMUNITY HEALTH NURSING?

Community health nursing differs from other kinds of practice in two important ways:

1. The unit of practice is the whole community.

2. The objective of practice is the promotion of health.

These two features—communities as clients and the focus on promoting health rather than managing disease—are related in important ways. Caring for the health of the public requires community-level intervention. By identifying a community's strengths and using those strengths as the starting place for protecting the health of citizens, community nurses have a profound influence on the health of individuals and families who live and work there.

The most essential and comprehensive community health nursing activity is enhancing community capacity (Kang, 1995). Community capacity is the extent to which local residents and institutions are equipped to manage the opportunities and problems the community is likely to confront. It is not unlike promoting the health of individuals and families so they can successfully manage the problems, losses, crises, and opportunities that are bound to occur over a lifetime. While there are many things outside their control, healthy communities can mobilize material and social resources to be ready for favorable and adverse trends and events so as to protect the growth and sustainability of community life. In places where there is an active citizen infrastructure, with a demonstrated capacity for community development and social planning, residents are able to reach a satisfactory resolution of health and social problems on their own (Cwikel, 1994).

WHAT IS A HEALTHY COMMUNITY?

The health of a community is not simply the aggregate of the health status of its individual citizens. Rather, it is a physical, economic, and social matrix that has the potential to fulfill the goals of *Healthy People 2010* (U.S. Department of Health and Human Services [USDHHS], 2001b).

- Extend the quality and years of healthy life for its citizens, and

- Eliminate health disparities.

Community health is less focused on individual health and access to personal health services and more on economic stability, educational opportunity, robust community institutions, citizen participation, and social justice. For example, Hornberger and Cobb (1998) found in their study of a rural Midwestern community that citizens valued the presence of a hospital and nursing home in their communities not so much because they provided accessible healthcare, but because these agencies provided jobs and economic stability for local residents. Respondents in the study cited kinship and other social relationships as well as community institutions (educational, religious, political) that facilitated a safe, caring environment for all citizens as indicators of a healthy community.

A community's health is the result of a complex interaction between the population and its environment. Using this ecological perspective, a community health problem reflects not just a problem with residents or a problem with the environment, but rather a problem with the relationship between them. To make it even more complex, human populations and environments change continuously; therefore, constant adaptation and readaptation are required to create and maintain healthy communities. Just as one health problem is resolved, new ones emerge to take its place. Milio (1975) put it succinctly: "Health is not a 'state' to be captured and dealt with; nor is it some achievement to be attained with finality. It is rather the response of people to their environment" (p. 3).

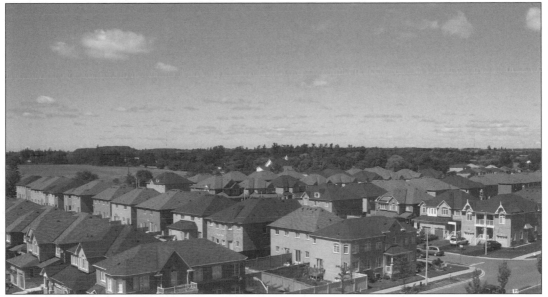

Photo by Farhan Amoor, Toronto, Ontario, Canada.

While this perspective suggests the quest for health, as an outcome, is futile, Dubos (1965) advised that while health is a goal that is ever changing, it is nonetheless one toward which we must continue to strive through new discoveries and new solutions to health problems.

In the world of reality, places change and man also changes. Further-more, his self-imposed striving for ever-new distant goals makes his fate even more unpredictable than that of other living things. For this reason, health and happiness cannot be absolute and permanent values, however careful the social and medical planning. Biological success in all its mani-festations is a measure of fitness, and fitness requires never-ending efforts of adaptation to the total environment, which is ever changing. (p. 29)

Health, as a constantly emerging relationship between populations and their physical and social environments, is easily grasped when common public health problems of the past, such as scurvy, smallpox, and polio, are compared with those of more recent years, such as motor vehicle accidents, drug abuse, school violence, nuclear disaster, terrorism, and, of course, HIV/AIDS (Gehlbach, 2005). Nevertheless, while new targets and objec-tives are established regularly, the overall goals of public health are basically unchanging. These include:

- Preserving a physical environment that supports human life,

- cultivating family and community support,

- enhancing each individual's inherent abilities to respond and to act, and

- assuring that all people achieve and maintain a maximum level of functioning, preventing premature death and preventing disability (USDHHS, 1990).

> It is not necessary for every citizen to know every other citizen or to share cultural beliefs and values, but the members of a community must have a kind and degree of intensity in their relationships with each other that distinguishes them from those outside the community.

WHAT IS A COMMUNITY?

What does the phrase "the community is the client" mean? The term *community* can be applied to almost any configuration of people whose common values, characteristics, and/or interests unite them in some way (e.g., a religious community, a retirement com-munity, or a community of scholars). While these are acceptable applications of the term community, they do not encompass the relationship between people and their habitat, which is the major concern of public health. Thus, for the purposes of community nursing, the concept of community must include:

- People (population),

- a physical place and time (environment) in which the population lives and works, and

- culture, or the ways in which citizens are organized and relate to each other and to their environment through shared beliefs, values, institutions, and social systems.

It is not necessary for every citizen to know every other citizen or to share cultural beliefs and values, but the members of a community must have a kind and degree of intensity in their relationships with each other that distinguishes them from those outside the community.

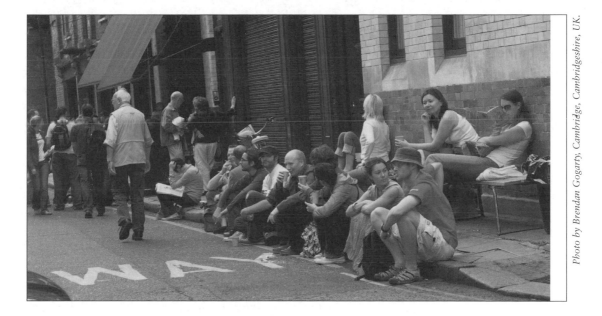

Photo by Brendan Gogarty, Cambridge, Cambridgeshire, UK.

POPULATION

Communities, of course, are made up of people, or populations. The term population simply refers to any category of people who share one or more designated characteristic (e.g., age, sex, eye color, residence, political orientation, occupation, disability, or religion). The population of a community, for example, would consist of all those individuals who share the common characteristic of residence in a designated place at a particular point in time. The population of Durham, NC, for example, is the aggregate number of people who reside within the established city boundaries of Durham at a particular moment in time. Unlike the more inclusive concept of community, a population is an objective reality and exactly equal to the sum of its parts. Thus, if the number of people residing in Gallup, NM, could be tabulated at a precise moment in time, it would be the same, no matter who measured it. In reality, of course, the size and characteristics of the population of Gallup (or any community) can change momentarily as residents are born, die, or migrate.

ENVIRONMENT

The second dimension of communities is location—the physical environment in which the population resides and interacts. The physical environment or context has two components: time and space. Communities not only occupy physical space, they occupy a place *in time*. Some communities may be very much like they were 100 years ago, while others have changed dramatically within the last 10 years. Communities have a history and a future that is highly relevant to community nursing practice. The interventions that worked 5, 10, or 20 years ago may no longer work today or tomorrow. The population may have changed from a young community to a retirement community or from an ethnically homogenous community to a highly diverse community. The quality of the physical environment is intrinsic to the health of the community, which is the expression of the relationship between a population and the environment.

> Although community is a more inclusive concept than population because it contains additional elements (culture and environment), it is possible for populations to include many communities and for communities to include many populations.

CULTURE

Although a community cannot exist without a population, a community is not just a collection of people occupying the same space at the same time. Community residents may go to school together, work for the same company, shop at the same store, attend the same churches, live in the same apartment building, or exercise at the same health club. The term community implies that there are social institutions that bring a population together in specific ways, at specific times, for specific purposes, such as religion, government, education, family groups, and commerce. Further, it implies the population must *relate* to its physical environment in discernable patterns and have identifiable rhythms of work, play, and domestic activity according to the day, week, and season. Finally, the term community indicates that there are values and social rules that guide the way people behave and interact with one another, and that these values and rules are passed through generations as part of learned behavior. All of these factors constitute the community's *culture* (Arensberg, 1961).

Communities represent the interaction of culture and environment. In this book, the term *culture* refers to the learned patterns of behavior and the range of beliefs and institutions attributed to a specific community. In most cases, individuals will have a limited impact on their cultural group or community, which has a life of its own and changes over time, independent of any one member. It is not necessary for the community's entire population to hold the same beliefs or share the same values or engage in the same behavior. As cultural groups, communities are composed of generations of families and individuals who enjoy varying levels of adherence to traditional cultural norms and values.

WHO IS THE CLIENT IN COMMUNITY HEALTH NURSING?

It should be clear by now that although they often are used interchangeably, communities and populations are not the same. Although community is a more inclusive concept than population because it contains additional elements (culture and environment), it is possible for populations to include many communities and for communities to include many populations. In reality, populations and communities are just different ways of looking at the same people. In community health practice, both population and community are used to monitor and protect the health of the public. It is critical, however, that we understand the difference. A community is not just the sum of its individual citizens.

POPULATIONS

Populations, which constitute the basic unit of analysis in epidemiology, are necessary for determining the health status of the public, identifying the magnitude of health problems, revealing the cause of disease and disability, and monitoring the effectiveness of public health action. Like K-12 education, maintaining roads, or providing protective services, public health is an official responsibility of government and therefore is generally organized according to geopolitical units such as counties, townships, municipalities, states, or nations. These geopolitical divisions are useful to governments that are held accountable for protecting the health of *all* citizens within them. Historically, throughout the world, public health departments have been responsible for safeguarding the health of whole populations in identified localities. This responsibility includes ongoing data collection, healthcare planning, and public health intervention.

The more entrepreneurial systems that characterize healthcare in the United States have designated loosely defined "catchment areas" and "market" populations as the units for service delivery. Furthermore, within the population of a designated health-delivery district (county, city, or catchment) there are any number of subpopulations (e.g., refugees, factory workers, people with lung cancer), each of which may have special health services and programs available through their companies, churches, foundations, and so on. Partnerships between private and public healthcare systems are increasingly common, but assurance that such partnerships have provided the necessary activities to protect the health of the entire citizenry (and not just those who have full or partial insurance) remains an official responsibility of public health agencies.

In recent health-systems terminology, the term *population-based* has been used to distinguish personal health services organized around a category based on disease or health needs of clients (the elderly, those with HIV/AIDS, pregnant women, children with chronic illness, etc.) from services organized according to a particular setting (intensive care, nursing home, inpatient, home health, etc.). The assumption is that these populations move in and out of settings depending on the services they need at a particular time; they are the same people but seen in different service areas. This definition is consistent with case management

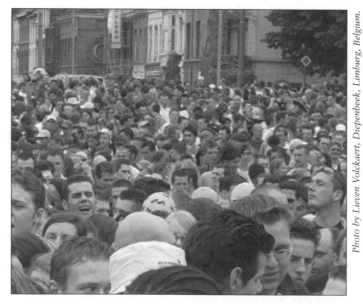

Photo by Lieven Volckaert, Diepenbeek, Limburg, Belgium.

programs and integrated systems of managed care. Thus, the *populations* of managed care systems are composed of the members of a particular healthcare plan. This differs significantly from public health practice in which the term *population-focused* signifies accountability for safeguarding the health of *all* people in a given locality, and not just individuals and families who currently are receiving services or who are enrolled in an insurance plan or a managed care program (Dreher, 1984).

COMMUNITIES

Unlike populations, which are concrete, communities are amorphous. They are not defined by external parameters such as political boundaries or disease categories. Rather, they are subjective and their definition—even of the same community—may vary from group to group or individual to individual. Thus, the same residentially based population could be described as a single community by a local politician, or as two communities by teachers working in its two school districts, or as several communities by members of various ethnic subpopulations. Although our public health conceptualization of community must include the three components of population, environment, and culture, the identification of a specific community is still subjective and may vary with the perspective of the identifier. For example, New York City officials may describe Manhattan Island as one community, representing one of the five boroughs that make up the city, but residents of Manhattan may identify many neighborhood communities, such as the Eastside, Tribeca, or Washington Heights. Still others may see the communities in terms of geographically based ethnic

communities such as Chinatown, Little Italy, or German Town. Because community boundaries, especially in urban environments, are likely to overlap and seldom are the same as geopolitical units, most public health services are organized according to geopolitically defined populations— rather than communities—to achieve accountability and comprehensiveness.

Even official, population-based health services are most effective, however, when they are designed and activated with the community in mind, because knowledge of the community is the vehicle through which the source of the problem and the cultural capital needed to fix it are identified. Take, for example, the *Healthy*

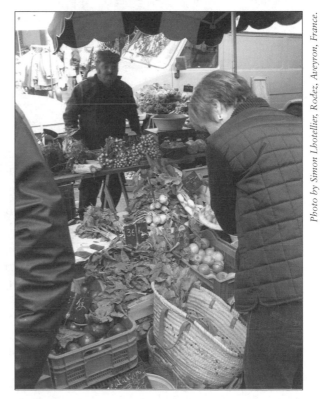

Photo by Simon Lhotellier, Rodez, Aveyron, France.

People 2010 objective to increase the rate of flu immunization coverage among adults 65 years of age and older to 90% (USDHHS, 2001b). To do this effectively, both population data and community cultural data are required. It would be important to know the number of cases of flu reported each year and the number of people immunized. At the very least, the size of the population of individuals over the age of 65 would need to be known to determine whether the 90% goal had been achieved. But, equally important is cultural knowledge about the position and status of elders (e.g., where they live, where they get together, how often they get together, for what purposes); basically, where do elders "fit" in community life? This information would help community health teams create the most

> Cultural knowledge helps us to predict and plan for the social and economic changes that will inevitably occur.

effective and efficient immunization program by utilizing the times and places in which elders in the community routinely come together—senior centers, local restaurants, libraries, religious centers, bingo games, golf courses, etc. The efficiencies inherent in such cultural knowledge also are likely to reduce costs while increasing participation in the program and perhaps even surpassing the 90% target.

BUILDING COMMUNITY CAPACITY THROUGH CULTURAL KNOWLEDGE

To determine the vision and hearing status of children between the ages of 10 and 14, it would not be necessary to identify and visit each house where children in that age range resided. Nor would it be appropriate to announce the availability of a screening program and hope that parents and children showed up. Instead, the program would be organized through the school system, where most children are conveniently gathered at predictable times. In addition, school records could be used to identify those children who were absent and required follow-up in order to assure evaluation of the entire population. Because schools are ongoing community institutions, once initiated, the program could be carried out routinely each year so that each child's performance could be traced over time, and if necessary, used to promote regulation to assure the schools would assume this responsibility each year.

While this example of schools as cultural capital seems almost self-evident, it is important to remember that each community, just like each individual, has distinct characteristics that must be identified and analyzed in a systematic and comprehensive assessment, incorporated into a community health agenda, and mobilized through culture-specific action. Thus parent-child community health practice is not just about providing personal health services in the form of prenatal care to a target population of high-risk mothers in prenatal clinics. Rather, it is about identifying the needs and problems of childbearing families in the community in relation to the social and economic fabric of community life. Cultural knowledge helps healthcare providers predict and plan for the social and economic changes that will inevitably occur.

Community health nurses who understand the trends and changes in the age and ethnic structure of the community's culture will be able to predict that in the next 5 years, the number of children under the age of 10 will increase dramatically; many of those children will come from families in which English is a second language; a substantial proportion of those children will be in need of day care while the mother is in the labor force; much of the care for children with health problems will be carried out by teachers and school nurses; and neighborhoods with the greatest influx of children may have safety and health hazards that will affect child welfare and development. Only with this kind of cultural knowledge can we create the optimal physical and social environments that will eliminate health disparities and extend the quality and years of healthy life for citizens (USDHHS, 2001a).

COMMUNITY NURSING PRACTICE

Taking care of a whole community is difficult to imagine and requires thinking about nursing in a different way. To better understand community health nursing, it is useful to compare the practice of the nurse engaged in the care of whole communities with that of the nurse "clinician" engaged in the care of individuals and families.

> Whereas the clinician interviews the patient, determining her age, ethnicity, residence, religion, occupation, and educational level, the community health nurse determines the sociodemographic characteristics of the population—age distribution, educational level, occupations, and so on.

ASSESSMENT AND ANALYSIS

Just as clinical practice begins with a systematic assessment of the individual client, community health nursing begins with a comprehensive and systematic assessment of the community client and its health problems (Rice, 1993). On entering the examining room, the clinician's first view of the patient includes head, torso, and extremities. Community health nurses, on entering a town, city, neighborhood, or county, may see major highways, a commercial center, schools, factories, government buildings, parks, perhaps a mountain range or prairie, a river dividing commercial areas, a residential suburb, recreational areas, and urban centers easing into farmland. Whereas the clinician interviews the patient, determining her age, ethnicity, residence, religion, occupation, and educational level, the community health nurse determines the sociodemographic characteristics of the population—age distribution, educational level, occupations, and so on. And while clinicians explore the organic and behavioral aspects of their patients and how they function and interrelate, community health nurses evaluate the community's social and economic institutions, class structures, neighborhood associations, ethnic groups, and the ways in which they function and interrelate (Arensberg, 1954).

In direct patient care, health status and health deviations are identified objectively through techniques such as physical examination and laboratory tests, and subjectively through taking a history and ascertaining the client's perspective on his or her health problem. Both objective and subjective findings are included in the analysis and diagnosis. In community health practice, inferences are drawn from demographic, sociological, environmental, and economic data sets, as well as from health status and health utilization data. Assessment tools include biostatistics, epidemiological studies, sociodemographic surveys, and community-based and household studies. Subjective data about the community include local definitions and commonly held values regarding health and illness. These can be obtained directly by talking with residents but also from the media, including radio, television, and local newspapers, as well as from observations of public behavior and community life.

With populations and communities as the primary units of nursing intervention, it is common to think in statistical terms when describing actual and potential health problems. This does not mean community health nurses have to be sophisticated mathematicians or perform complex statistical analyses. Rather, it means community health nurses must think in terms of rates, patterns, and trends. For example, an individual patient either has or does not have heart disease, but a population has a rate of heart disease that may compare favorably or unfavorably with the rate of heart disease in another population or in a previous time period for that population. Similarly, a woman is either pregnant or she is not pregnant, but in community health nursing it is possible for a community to be "a little bit" pregnant or "a lot" pregnant. Though many shudder at the mention of statistics, such quantitative findings are the lab results that help healthcare professionals diagnose the health of communities and demonstrate the influence of community health nurses on health and on the lives of hundreds of thousands of people. It is exciting to be able to show dramatic changes in the rates or patterns of diabetes as a result of a community diet and exercise program. It is deeply satisfying to use statistical comparisons of populations to predict that some neighborhoods are at greater risk for drug abuse or to demonstrate how after-school programs in the junior high schools have decreased teenage pregnancy and high school dropout rates.

> Community health nursing, on the other hand, requires different kinds of nursing interventions that include public speaking, journalistic writing, social marketing, record keeping, statistical analysis, program development and evaluation, political action, and policy formulation and administration.

COMMUNITY PLANNING AND INTERVENTION

After assessing the patient and determining a diagnosis, clinicians integrate patient and provider goals, assuring that the plan is culturally acceptable, as well as clinically appropriate. Intervention strategies may include both social and individual adjustments. For example, several objectives in *Healthy People 2010* are focused on the reduction of asthma, which is currently one of the top 10 reasons for emergency room visits in the United States. Direct medical expenditures for asthma were more than $3.6 billion, with another $2.6 billion in indirect economic losses (USDHHS, 2001b). The care plan for a patient with asthma is likely to include breathing and relaxation exercises, inhalation therapy, one-to-one teaching, family counseling, and an emergency action plan. In contrast, the asthma care plan for a community may include identification of vulnerable populations, implementation of screening programs, utilization of media resources for health education, implementation of smoking cessation programs in schools and workplaces, formulation of public policies on air pollution levels, and organization of community action groups to control industrial wastes.

Personal health services require diverse nursing procedures such as therapeutic counseling, vital sign assessments, aseptic techniques, medication, and/or patient education. These procedures, among countless others, are the stock and trade of the clinician. Activities such as counseling a parent, changing a dressing, putting a patient through range of motion exercises, irrigating a catheter, or teaching a family member how to administer insulin are easily identified as nursing care. Community health nursing, on the other hand, requires different kinds of nursing interventions that include public speaking, journalistic writing, social marketing, record keeping, statistical analyses, program development and evaluation, political action, policy formulation, and administration. When the community is the client, interventions take place at the community level. They might include, for example, promoting legislation to mandate the presence of school health nurses, being interviewed on a Spanish radio program, writing a guest column on how to select a nursing home, mobilizing support for the clean-up of toxic waste, or collecting data on the number of cases of sexually transmitted infections (STIs) in a specific community.

Clinicians and community health nurses often use the same kinds of interventions, such as education, but apply it differently. For example, after assessing the patient's knowledge, peri-operative nurses provide individualized post-surgical instructions so the patient can be informed of what to expect, what to do, where to go, and whom to ask in the event of an emergency. This education relieves anxiety, encourages rehabilitation, prevents complications, hastens recovery, and engages the patient in a therapeutic plan of care. Community health nurses, on the other hand, accountable for community-wide disaster preparedness, may discover that while there is a carefully formulated disaster plan, the majority of community residents are unaware of it. To assure the community is knowledgeable and prepared for a disaster, community health nurses may engage the assistance of community agencies, including schools, radio stations, and the chamber of commerce; publish the plan in local news media; establish periodic disaster drills; enlist and educate volunteers; and work with local merchants to create a "disaster list" of food, water, batteries, candles, and so on, to assure that all members and sectors of the community are informed and ready.

Coordination is another nursing responsibility that is played out differently in clinical practice and community health practice. One of the responsibilities of nurse clinicians is to coordinate the services of the physician, social worker, radiologist, physical therapist, lab technician, and so on, so patient care unfolds in a way that is both therapeutic and efficient. In comparison, the community health nurse is responsible for identifying community resources (cultural capital) and determining how these resources can be integrated and deployed to promote the health of the community. This might include, for example, bringing religious leaders of different denominations together to improve the quality of life for elderly members of the community or working with major industries to develop child health and day-care programs for working parents. In the political arena, community health nurses may bring legislators, industrial leaders, and emission experts together to create policies that will improve the air quality of communities. Community nurses work in partnership with local organizations, media resources, and influential community leaders to create healthy communities.

EVALUATION

The effectiveness of direct patient care is determined by assessing the degree to which it is successful in achieving the outcomes that have been established by the client and the nurse. This could include recovering from an illness, becoming alcohol-free, reducing emergency room visits for a child with asthma, having an uncomplicated birth experience, or having a peaceful and meaningful death. Efficiency and cost enter the evaluation process as the nurse determines whether the same outcomes can be achieved at less cost, or better outcomes can be achieved at the same cost.

In community health nursing, the desired outcome is the extent to which certain activities have strengthened capacity and achieved a healthier community—a place that is safer, cleaner, and more tolerant; where people live longer, more productive, and happier lives; and where health disparities have been eliminated. In community health practice, evaluation must also include assessing whether the correct initiatives are being implemented to create a healthier community. A successful anti-smoking campaign, for example, may reduce tobacco consumption among teenagers but may have little effect on assuring the health of the community, because local industry has not been persuaded to comply with recommended clean-air emission standards.

THE NURSE-CLIENT RELATIONSHIP

The comparisons presented thus far suggest compelling differences in the nurse-client relationship when the move is from individual clients to community clients. Unlike most areas of practice in which nurses see a relatively small and select category of patients—usually under very special circumstances—community health nurses work with the whole population in the everyday circumstances of community life. As such, community health nurses should be highly visible, taking part in community events and making themselves known to all sectors of the community and its various leaders. Through reputation and relationships, influence is cultivated to support community health programs and policy reform. Relationships with individuals and groups and knowledge of the community's cultural capital are essential in detecting and solving community problems.

Although all nurses are, consciously or unconsciously, role models for their clients, role modeling is particularly important for community health nurses. Constantly under the scrutiny of community residents, community health nurses exemplify, in appearance and behavior, the expectations set for community residents in terms of healthy behavior and public service. This is especially critical in the area of prevention and health promotion. How can community health nurses launch a campaign to eliminate cigarette smoking in all public places if they are smokers? How do community health nurses convince high school administrators to initiate nutrition education programs if they have poor dietary habits? And how do community health nurses encourage citizens to vote and engage in public service, unless they are active participants in community public life?

There is also the matter of confidentiality. Therapeutic relationships, grounded in trust and mutual respect, are essential for effective intervention in every nursing situation. This is no less significant, but perhaps more complicated, in community intervention, where the focus of practice is an entire community of people, some of whom may be at odds with one another or, at the very least, curious and cautious about one another. The betrayal of confidence with just one resident or community organization can generate a community-wide lack of trust and easily compromise effectiveness.

Unlike individual clients, communities are composed of many individuals and diverse groups who may have competing problems and conflicting goals and priorities. To be a potent force in achieving the public's health requires setting aside personal or group loyalties and working for the benefit of the community as a whole. Desired outcomes are accomplished through coordination and articulation of community constituents and through development of "win-win" strategies. To do this, community health nurses must know the various groups and factions of the community, all of which must have—and know that they have—equal access to and the consideration of the community health nurse.

Finally, the timing and cycles of activity in community health practice are different from those of clinical practice. First of all, community health nursing is necessarily future-oriented, engaging in interventions now so as to avert problems that are likely to occur in 5 or 10 years. For example, good community health practice is sensitive to the profound changes that a young immigrant group will bring to a community. These might include increased fertility rates, younger mothers, higher parity, and beliefs and practices related to child development that will require modification in child care, education, and health services. Second, things happen much more slowly in community health nursing. Unlike direct patient care, where laboratory tests can be performed, reported, and acted upon in a matter of hours or even minutes, it often takes months, years, or decades to detect changes and trends in the health status of a community. The lapse between an intervention and its outcomes may be frustrating for those who like to see immediate results. For example, a teenage-parent education program may not demonstrate a community-wide decrease in child abuse for 3 to 5 years after the program is conceived and initiated. This requires patience and accurate records in order to trace patterns of health, disease, and sociodemographic changes. Unlike a patient care plan, comprehensive planning for the community's health is not something that is undertaken and completed within a specific health event. Rather, it is an ongoing, routine part of community nursing practice. Thus, 5- and 10-year plans, usually revised annually, serve as a guide to the daily, weekly, and monthly activities of the community health nurse.

The future and long-range orientation of community health practice poses some interesting dilemmas, because the real measure of effectiveness is not how well problems are handled as they occur, but how successfully crises are averted or managed. It is difficult to assess the quality of community health nursing, because it may be based on events that do not happen. Likewise, it is not easy to engage community enthusiasm for avoiding problems that are unlikely to occur for many years, if ever. On the other hand, the magnitude of the results in terms of the hundreds, thousands, and even millions of people affected now and in the future can be thrilling for those fascinated by the opportunity to build sustainable communities, reshape healthcare, and ameliorate large-scale health problems.

COMMUNITY NURSING VALUES AND CONFLICTS

The fact that communities are composed of groups with conflicting goals and competing values creates profound ethical issues in public health practice. Indeed, one of the most distinguishing features of community health nursing is its value orientation, in which the community's goals take precedence over those of the individual in identifying and achieving the "common good" (Mechanic, 1998; Winkelstein, 1996). The public health practitioner, whose practice may include both direct and community-based care, often is caught in a web of competing values. This tension between individual and society in assuring the public's health has always existed. Freeman (1963), an early leader in community health nursing education in the United States, addressed this dilemma:

> The selection of those to be served ... must rest on the comparative
> impact on community health rather than solely on the needs of the individ-

ual or family being served. ... The community health nurse cannot elect to care for a small number of people intensely while ignoring the needs of many others. She must be concerned with the community as a whole. (p. 35)

This passage leaves no room for doubt. When there is conflict between individual goals and community goals, community goals must prevail. Such conflicts typically arise when there is competition for limited health resources. For example, consider a community in which a small number of individuals could benefit by the presence of sophisticated cardiology technology in a local hospital. The families of these individuals and their cardiologists may present a strong case for having these procedures available locally. On the other hand, the community may achieve more enduring, less costly, and better outcomes if resources were directed toward prevention rather than disease management; for example, a community-based cardiac health education program to instruct all families in the community on the principles of good cardiac health.

> One of the most distinguishing features of community health nursing is its value orientation, in which the community's goals take precedence over those of the individual in identifying and achieving the "common good."

There are times when community health nurses may have to select among competing values for the good of the whole. Formulating a plan of action that is consistent with the goals of both the larger community and the expectations of individual clients and families often is difficult to achieve. Communities are complex aggregates, and while some values are shared among all residents, groups within the community may hold opposing values that usually are expressed around particular issues and events. Thus, not only are there bound to be occasions of conflict between individual and community-level objectives, but also, as has already been pointed out, among different factions within communities (Bibeau, 1997).

With these opposing demands, how is the common good defined? The good of the whole community does not necessarily mean the desires of the majority. Imagine, for example, a community in which a particular industry (which happens to be the largest employer of community residents) is engaged in a conflict with the health department and concerned citizens regarding its dangerous waste-disposal practices. If compliance with waste-disposal regulations has economic consequences for employees, such as reductions in workforce or decreased wages, it is likely the industry will have the majority of the population among its supporters, with only a few advocating for a more enduring approach to public health.

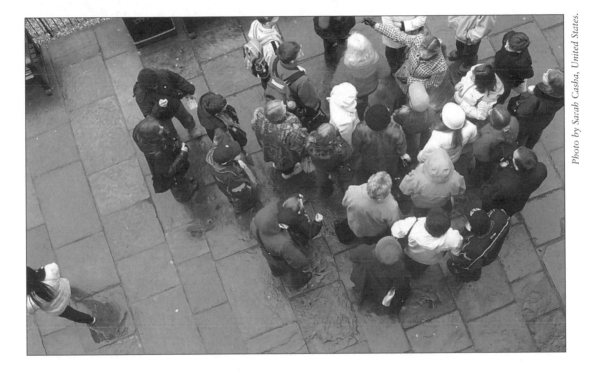

Photo by Sarah Casha, United States.

Caring for the health of the public requires not only a shift in the practice paradigm, but also a shift in the values that influence priority-setting and decision-making when faced with the inevitable conflict between individual and public health and among special interest stakeholders within communities. The way in which community health nursing resources (e.g., time, expertise, funding, and influence) are deployed must be reflective of the whole community now and in the future.

COMMUNITY HEALTH NURSING: A WORK IN PROGRESS

Before leaving this introduction to community health nursing, it is useful to review the evolution of this kind of nursing practice and speculate on its future. The tradition for public health nursing was established in Liverpool, England, during the Victorian age with the support of William Rathbone, a wealthy merchant and social reformer. On the advice of Florence Nightingale, Rathbone opened a training school in 1862 to prepare "district nurses" who would oversee the health of designated communities. Meanwhile, American nursing activists, with the assistance of prominent women who had been to England and were strongly influenced by the work of Rathbone and Nightingale, began to institute district nursing in the United States. By the time Lillian Wald established the Henry Street Settlement in New York City in the 1890s, district nursing organizations had already been established in other cities.

These community health services, modeled after those in Great Britain, were available to the entire population in a designated area. The emphasis on prevention was clearly recognized by Wald, who contended that all people, whether sick or ill, should receive health services (Buhler-Wilkerson, 1993). In addition to a home nursing service, Wald established a school nurse program to attend to the health needs of school-age children and their families. "Universal" service became the hallmark of district nursing. Based on these early examples scattered through the major cities of the United States, district nursing also was brought to rural areas, mainly through the efforts of voluntary organizations such as the American Red Cross.

After the turn of the century, there was a marked shift toward specialization in public health nursing, prompted by a trend toward disease-oriented funding programs, such as tuberculosis control or detection and management of STIs. Formerly generalists, district nurses took on specialized roles in the care of individuals with particular health problems. Universal service, the birthright of community nurses, was gradually relinquished, and generalized practice was replaced by an increasing concentration on special programs, such as maternal child health and communicable disease control. Whether community health nurses should be generalists or specialists has been debated for many decades. Those who prefer specialized roles cite cost-saving features and higher quality of care as major benefits. Those favoring the generalist approach, on the other hand, contend that community health nurses are there to promote the health of the whole community and not just serve the needs of those with specific diseases or problems. They argue, moreover, that the development of many categorical programs confuses clients and, far from reducing costs, results in expensive duplication of services.

In many places, the titles *public health nurse* and *community health nurse* came to mean any nursing activity that was located outside of a hospital setting. Thus, the "community" in community health nursing took on significance as the practice *setting*, rather than the practice *orientation* and unit of services. In recent years, the shift of acute care from the hospital to the home has created even more confusion about the role and definition of community health nurses.

In nursing education, similar changes were taking place. Once the hallmark of a bachelor's degree in nursing, community health nursing, in its purest sense, was reserved for the final semesters. As the culminating generalist experience, it subsumed and synthe sized all the various areas of nursing previously learned at the individual and family levels of practice. In subsequent years, however, new curricula integrated the community experi ence with parent-child nursing, psychiatric nursing, geriatric nursing, and so on, so that the role of community or public health nursing in safeguarding the health of whole com munities was even further obscured.

As a response to the changes taking place in practice and education, the 1970s and 1980s saw a revival of interest in trying to understand and differentiate public and com munity health nursing from other kinds of nursing practice. Many experts expressed con cern about the lack of definition in public health nursing and looked for ways to reintro duce its principles into nursing education curricula (Roberts & Freeman, 1973; Skrovan, Anderson, & Gottschalk, 1974). They cautioned the visiting nurse's *caseload* should *not* be confused with the public health *district*, which includes all people—well and ill. Williams (1977) identified the major problems in distinguishing community health nurs ing from other areas of nursing practice. They included (1) the propensity to define com munity health nursing based on the setting in which it takes place rather than on the focus of practice, and (2) the lack of healthcare programs and settings where nurses can engage in a true community health or public health practice.

In 1980, responding to the growing concern over the failure to delineate the unique ness of public and community health nursing, both the American Nurses Association (ANA) and the Public Health Nursing Section of the American Public Health Association (APHA) issued definitive statements. According to the American Nurses Association (1980),

> Community health nursing is a synthesis of nursing practice and public health practice applied to promoting and preserving the health of com munities. The practice is general and comprehensive. It is not limited to a particular age group or diagnosis, and is continuing, not episodic. The dominant responsibility is to the community as a whole. (p. 2)

A similar position was taken by the APHA (1980) in the statement from the Public Health Nursing Section:

> Public health nursing synthesizes the body of knowledge from the public health sciences and professional nursing theories for the purpose of improving the health of the entire community. This goal lies at the heart of primary prevention and health promotion and is the foundation for

> public health nursing practice. ... In summary, the specialty of public
> health nursing is professional nursing directed toward a total community
> or community group. Consideration is given to environmental, social,
> and personal health factors affecting health status. Emphasis is on plan-
> ning for a community as a whole rather than on individual health care.

These statements were bold departures from earlier definitions in which the family,
rather than the community, was the unit of service and the setting (sociodemographic)
was offered as the major defining feature of community health nursing. In spite of the
increasing emphasis on communities as the unit of service delivery and the defining feature of public health nursing, however, both ANA and APHA statements continued to see
personal health services as a major vehicle through which community health could be
obtained. For example, in the ANA (1980) definition:

> Nursing directed to individuals, families, or groups contributes to the
> health of the total community. Health promotion, health maintenance,
> health education, and management, coordination, and continuity of care
> are utilized in a holistic approach to the management of the healthcare of
> individuals, families and groups in a community.

Similarly, the Public Health Nursing Section definition suggested that, in order to
accomplish community health goals, "community health nurses work with groups, families,
and individuals as well as in multidisciplinary teams and programs" (APHA, 1980).

In 1984, the Division of Nursing, U.S. Department of Health and Human Services
(Bureau of Health Professions of the Health Resources and Services Administration) sponsored a national consensus conference titled "Essentials of Public Health Nursing Practice
and Education," in collaboration with the American Nurses Association, the American
Public Health Association, and other nursing organizations (USDHHS, 1984). The goals
of this conference were to agree upon the direction of community health or public health
nursing and identify the educational preparation needed to practice as both a generalist
and a specialist. In debating the definitions of community and community health nursing,
expert nurses from both practice and education still could not relinquish the focus on
personal health services to individuals and families.

> Public health nurses are concerned primarily with health promotion,
> health maintenance, and health education and with the coordination of
> healthcare in the community. They promote the well being of individuals
> and families and seek to foster continuity of care within the community.
> The distinguishing characteristic of the service they provide is its focus on

the health needs of specific community groups, especially those most vulnerable or those who are at risk of disease or disability. (p. 7)

Not until recently have the definitions of public health nursing, forwarded by the ANA and the Public Health Nursing Section of the APHA, emphasized populations as the centerpiece of public health practice. In addition, they have qualified the role of nurses providing care to individuals and families. The ANA (1996) Scope and Standards of Population-Focused, Community-Oriented Nursing Practice made the distinction between population-focused and community-based care in defining public health nursing:

> Population-focused or public health nursing is defined by the nature of its responsibility to all of the people, the partnership with the people and the emergence of programs and activities from a systematic assessment process. Nurses who are focused on the care of individuals or families are essential to the provision of population-focused nursing services, for they contribute to improving the health of entire populations. That contribution is not sufficient or comprehensive enough to be defined as population-focused nursing practice, for it does not aid in distinguishing the specialty of population-focused nursing practice from other forms of nursing practice. (p. 3)

In this model, personal health services to individuals and families fall under the category of "assurance activities." This includes those activities that are necessary to promote the health of communities by safeguarding the health of all individuals and families—usually those who put the entire population at risk and whose personal healthcare is not provided by any other organization.

The statement submitted by the Public Health Nursing Section of APHA (1996) also emphasizes *populations* in its basic definition and de-emphasizes the provision of personal health services except for assurance activities.

> The title "public health nurse" designates a nursing professional with educational preparation in public health and nursing science with a primary focus on community-level outcomes. The primary focus of public health nursing is to promote health and prevent disease for entire population groups. This may include assisting and providing care to individual members of the population. It also includes the identification of individuals who may not request care but who have health problems that put themselves and others in the community at risk, such as those with infectious diseases. The focus of public health nursing is not on providing

direct care to individuals in community settings. Public health nurses support the provision of direct care through a process of evaluation and
assessment of the needs of individuals in the context of their population
group. Public health nurses work with other providers of care to plan,
develop and support systems and programs in the community to prevent
problems and provide access to care. (p. 2)

Unfortunately, neither the ANA nor the APHA description regarded the community
as the actual *client,* but rather as the *context* for the delivery of personal health services
or for the development of programs and systems of care.

Community-based care is defined ... as care that is provided outside of
an institution (in the community). This care is primarily provided to individuals and families. (ANA, 1996, p. 4)

Public health nurses work with other providers of care to plan, develop
and support systems and programs in the community to prevent problems and provide access to care. (APHA, 1996, p. 2)

In the most recent draft of the ANA (2005) Scope and Standards of Public Health Nursing
Practice, intended to replace the 1986 Standards of Community Health Nursing, the focus
is almost exclusively on populations with only secondary reference to communities as the
target of nursing intervention. This discounting of community as client may be attributable
to the way in which the ANA (2005) defines community without reference to culture, as "a
group of people who have common characteristics ... defined by location, race, ethnicity,
age, occupation, interest in particular problems or outcomes, or other common bonds"
(p. 55). Although the Quad Council of Public Health Nursing Organizations (QCPHNO;
2004) clearly defined the community dimensions of public health practice, it did not take
the concept of culture much beyond the issue of diversity and cultural competence.

More recently, the influence of managed care and its companion vernacular has
added confusion and, to some extent, compromised official definitions of community
health nursing. The attempt to clarify the scope of public health nursing practice by the
QCPHNO (1999) reflects this problem.

Some public health nurses may have responsibility for the health of a
geographic or enrolled population, such as those covered by a health
department or capitated health system, whereas others may promote the
health of a specific population, for example, those with HIV/AIDS. (p. 2)

Although this description captures most of the major tenets of public health, its inclusion of enrolled members in a capitated health plan as a focus of intervention compromises one of the most fundamental tenets of public health, e.g., health protection for the *entire* public. Nurses' responsibility for the health of enrollees in a capitated health system may be population-based, but it is not public health (Bender & Salmon, 2001).

Some may argue with what might be considered an overly purist definition of public and community health, grounded in the philosophical underpinnings of *Health for All*, coined at Alma Ata (World Health Organization, 1979), as well as the *Healthy People* Series.

Nursing continues to struggle with the definitions and titles that will most significantly impact the professional charged with promoting the public's health through work with communities and populations (Drevdahl, 1995). Although the debate is understandable, no position is taken by the authors on whether *community health nurse* or *public health nurse* should be the official title. In this book, both terms are used interchangeably and situationally. The obvious preference for *community nurse*, however, reflects the cultural orientation of this book, which necessitates attention to communities, and the conviction that it is communities, not populations, with which nurses engage to promote and sustain the public's health.

> Public health, however, implies not just a commitment to the health of specific populations, but a social responsibility for the health of all citizens in all communities, states, nations, and the world.

The most effective resolution of large-scale health problems, throughout history, continues to be accomplished not through individual patient care, but through intervention at the community level, in political, economic, and social arenas (Koop, 1995; Milio, 1975). The culturally grounded approach advocated in this book is a blueprint for such intervention, for it is in the naturally occurring laboratories of communities that the conditions of health, as opposed to the causes of illness, are most likely to be found. Given the increasing confirmation, for example, that the key to health and reduced morbidity and mortality lies in the capacity of communities to invest all of its citizens in local life, it is interesting how much of community nursing practice continues to focus exclusively on medical interventions (immunization, mammograms, physical check-ups, screening procedures) and how little on community relationship-building. How many family practice clinicians—physicians or nurse practitioners—for example, include enhancement of social networks as part of their therapy, as opposed to prescribing antidepressants to make lonely people at least functional? Improving the health of the public is not limited to advances in medical science and technology, but rather encompasses an infinite range of activities, many of which are outside the so-called "healthcare system." For example, a mother's education has been identified as a significant predictor of neonatal health and development (Rubinstein & Lane, 1990), yet how many resources are invested in educating women in third-world countries, compared with that invested in pediatric services, pharmaceuticals, and equipment? Self-help movements such as Alcoholics Anonymous, Weight Watchers, and cancer survivor groups also provide compelling evidence of the value of a social model of healthcare.

It is time to renew a commitment to traditional public health values to assure that all citizens of communities—whether they are sick or well, insured or uninsured—have a safe and healthy place in which to live, work, play, and raise families. Culturally competent healthcare begins with inclusiveness and the engagement of all community members and organizations and culminates in eliminating health disparities and prolonging the years of healthy life for all populations. *Public health has never been more important.* In the chapters that follow, the reader will discover how to work at the systems level, using the concept of culture to accomplish the kind and magnitude of change that will truly improve the health of the public. The authors will explore the principles of community health practice that begin with assessing communities, then move to the identification of current and potential community problems, and ultimately to the development of culture-specific solutions.

REFERENCES

American Nurses Association. (1980). *Standards of community health nursing practice.* Washington, DC: Author.

American Nurses Association. (1996). *Scope and standards of community-focused, community-oriented nursing practice.* Washington, DC: Author.

American Nurses Association. (2005). *Public health nursing: Scope and standards of practice.* Draft document.

American Public Health Association. (1980, June). *The definition and role of public health nursing in the delivery of health care: A position paper by the Public Health Nursing Section* (Working Draft III). Washington, DC: Author.

American Public Health Association. (1996). *The definition and role of public health nursing: A statement of APHA.* Washington, DC: Author.

Arensberg, C. (1954). The community study method. *American Journal of Sociology, 60*(2), 109-124.

Arensberg, C. (1961). Community as object and as sample. *American Anthropology, 63,* 241-264.

Bender, K.W., & Salmon, M.E. (2001). Public health nursing: Pioneers of health care reform. In K.S. Lundy & S. Janes (Eds.), *Community health nursing: Caring for the public's health* (pp. 866-877). Boston: Jones & Bartlett.

Bibeau, G. (1997). At work in the fields of public health: The abuse of rationality. *Medical Anthropology Quarterly, 11*(2), 246-252.

Buhler-Wilkerson, K. (1993). Bringing care to the people: Lillian Wald's legacy to public health nursing. *American Journal of Public Health, 83*(12), 1778-1786.

Cwikel, J.G. (1994). After epidemiological research: What next? Community action for health promotion. *Public Health Revues, 22,* 375-394.

Dreher, M. (1984). District nursing: The cost-benefits of a community-based practice. *American Journal of Public Health, 74*(10), 1107-1111.

Drevdahl, D. (1995). Coming to voice: The power of emancipatory community interventions. *Advances in Nursing Science, 18*(2), 13-24.

Dubos, R. (1965). *Man adapting.* New Haven, CT: Yale University Press.

Freeman, R. (1963). *Public health nursing practice* (3rd ed.). Philadelphia: Saunders.

Gehlbach, S. (2005). *American plagues: Lessons from our battles with disease.* New York: McGraw Hill.

Hornberger, C., & Cobb, A. (1998). A rural vision of a healthy community. *Public Health Nursing, 15*(5), 363-369.

Kang, R. (1995). Building community capacity for health promotion: A challenge for public health nurses. *Public Health Nursing, 12*(5), 312-318.

Koop, C.E. (1995). Editorial: A personal role in health care reform. *American Journal of Public Health, 85*(6), 759-760.

Mechanic, D. (1998). Topics for our times: Managed care and public health opportunities. *American Journal of Public Health, 88*(6), 874-875.

Milio, N. (1975). *The care of health in communities.* New York: Macmillan.

Quad Council of Public Health Nursing Organizations. (1999). *Scope and standards of public health nursing practice.* Washington, DC: American Nurses Publishing.

Quad Council of Public Health Nursing Organizations. (2004). Public health nursing competencies. *Public Health Nursing, 21*(5), 443-452.

Rice, J.A. (1993). Community health assessment. The first step in community health planning. *Hospital Technology Series, 12*(13), 1-32.

Roberts, D.E., & Freeman, R.B. (1973). *Redesigning nursing education for public health* (DHEW Publication NO. 75-75). Washington, DC: U.S. Government Printing Office.

Rubinstein, R.A., & Lane, S.D. (1990). International health and development. In T.M. Johnson & C.F. Sargent (Eds.), *Medical Anthropology* (pp. 367-390). Westport, CT: Praeger Press.

Skrovan, C., Anderson, E.T., & Gottschalk, J. (1974, September). Community nurse practitioner: An emerging role. *American Journal of Public Health, 64,* 847-853.

U.S. Department of Health and Human Services. (1984). *Consensus conference on the essentials of public health nursing practice and education* (Report of Conference September 5-7). Rockville, MD: Author.

U.S. Department of Health and Human Services. (1990). *Healthy people 2000: National health promotion and disease prevention objectives.* Washington, DC: Government Printing Office.

U.S. Department of Health and Human Services. (2001a). *Cultural competence works. Using cultural competence to improve the quality of health care for diverse populations and add value to managed care arrangements.* (Government publications 98-0372). Merrifield, VA: Author.

U.S. Department of Health and Human Services. (2001b). *Healthy people 2010.* McLean, VA: International Medical Publishing.

Williams, C. (1977). Community health nursing—What is it? *Nursing Outlook, 25,* 250-254.

Winkelstein, W. (1996). Editorial: Eras, paradigms, and the future of epidemiology. *The American Journal of Public Health, 86*(5), 621-622.

World Health Organization. (1979). *Formulating strategies for health for all by the year 2000: Guiding principles and essential issues.* Geneva, Switzerland: Author.

CULTURE AND HEALTH ASSESSMENT FOR COMMUNITY HEALTH PRACTICE

In the next two chapters, the basic information necessary to describe and analyze a community's health is presented. As *Healthy People 2010* makes abundantly clear, many aspects of a community's culture, identified in Chapter 3, can determine its health status—rules that govern family and social life, ideas about health and illness, educational opportunities and religious affiliation, poverty and conversely wealth, adequacy of housing and sanitation, age distribution, availability of health statistics, and commitment to eliminating health disparities, to mention only a few. The health beliefs, problems, behaviors, and systems addressed in Chapter 4 constitute only one aspect of a community's culture. Thus, while they are presented in separate chapters, cultural assessment and health assessment are inextricably related.

The framework for the assessment of both culture and health underscores the importance of a community's history and environment as a place in time, the shift from individual and family to community clients or populations, and the way each community's social system affects health. These three approaches to understanding how communities work enable intelligent and responsible community practice for promoting the public's health. Acting to assure children can walk safely to school requires an understanding of economic, political, and moral imperatives in contemporary community life and the prevailing social beliefs around individual and social responsibility.

Compared to assessing an individual patient, the health of a population and environment and the cultural capital a social system directs to the health of a community are necessarily a complicated business that draws from both the social sciences, such as anthropology and political science, and the biological sciences that gird public health. Ethnography and epidemiology combine to create the most comprehensive assessment of culture, health, and community.

Since a community's health is the result of a complex interaction between the population and its environment, a community health assessment must include both the population and the environment. The impact of the environment on the current and future health of the community is obvious—regulation of smoking in public places, sanitary conditions in restaurants, clean air, clean water, and fire protection are all functions that have an obvious impact on improving the environment in which citizens reside. The health status of a population is more obscure, and there often is a tension between what constitutes a personal health problem and a public health problem. This tension is often manifest in the unique social organization found in each community.

Nevertheless, while new targets and objectives are established each decade by the *Healthy People Series,* the overall goals of public health are basically unchanging. They include preserving a physical environment that supports human life, cultivating family and community support, enhancing each individual's inherent abilities to respond and to act, assuring that all persons achieve and maintain a maximum level of functioning, preventing premature death, and preventing disability (U.S. Department of Health and Human Services, [USDHHS], 1990).

References

U.S. Department of Health and Human Services. (1990). *Healthy people 2000: National health promotion and disease prevention objectives.* Washington, DC: Government Printing Office.

CHAPTER

COMMUNITY CULTURAL ASSESSMENT

Culture is not just about ethnicity. Rather, it is about a community's use of space and time, its life ways, and the manner in which its people are organized.

In Chapter 2, health was conceptualized as the ongoing expression of the relationship between humans and their physical and social environments. The focus of community health nursing, therefore, is not just people but the interaction between people and their environments. This interaction constitutes the culture of community—the blueprint for daily life. A cultural assessment identifies the community's resources, or the cultural capital, necessary for achieving the two goals of *Healthy People 2010:* eliminating health disparities and increasing the quality and years of healthy life (U.S. Department of Health and Human Services [USDHHS], 2001).

CHAPTER 3 OBJECTIVES

- Identify the sources and methods of data gathering about the cultural capital of a community.

- Describe the spatial and temporal dimensions of community life that impact on health and health services.

- Delineate the sociodemographic characteristics of populations that are significant for determining community health status.

- Identify the major components of social organization that impact on health and healthcare.

- Apply the methods for analyzing cultural assessment data to formulating a healthy community agenda.

Community assessment is the foundation for community nursing practice (American Public Health Association, 1996; Quad Council of Public Health Nursing Organizations, 2004). Culture mediates all aspects of community life, including health behaviors and institutions. Culture is not just about ethnicity. Rather, it is about a community's use of space and time, its life ways (e.g., family structure, work patterns, education, religion, recreation, etc.), and the manner in which its people are organized. Thus, the concept of community embraces three different, but interrelated, perspectives:

- a place in time,

- a population, and

- a social organization.

The data collection instrument that forms the basis for community health assessment in this chapter is a traditional approach to the study of communities developed by cultural anthropologist Conrad Arensberg (1954). This method of data gathering is known as ethnography. Originally developed in the discipline of anthropology, it has been used extensively by the nursing profession (Munhall, 2002; Schultz & Magilvy, 1988; Schulte, 2000). For decades, this method—or variations of it—has been used to describe cultures by examining human behavior in the context of community. As the role of anthropologists has shifted from a broad exploration of culture to the exploration of contemporary social problems, anthropologists have not had the luxury of spending months or even years of total immersion in the field. In response to this shift in roles, the last decades have seen the development of several rapid assessment techniques (Chambers, 1985; Clark et al., 2003; Ervin, 1997; Needle et al., 2003; Scrimshaw & Hurtado, 1987) that employ field teams, focus groups, and other more directed forms of inquiry about specific problems. Such guides are still grounded in standard ethnographic methods, however, and the objective is still a comprehensive assessment of the community's culture.

Although it looks quite extensive, the format for cultural assessment that follows is not exhaustive. First, it attempts to identify the range of information a community health nurse would find useful for successful community health practice. Second, it provides a simple but meaningful way to organize cultural information into categories so inferences can easily be drawn. This tool is intended for use in all kinds of communities—rural, urban, agricultural, tourist, large, small, middle class, working class—and for communities in less technologically developed societies, as well as in industrialized societies. Therefore, some of the questions and categories may not apply to every community, or they may seem self-evident. The important thing is *not* the completion of every category of the instrument, but rather the collection and management of community information. It encompasses the broad categories highlighted in *Healthy People 2010* as accounting for health disparities in the United States: gender, race and ethnicity, income and education, disability, rural localities, and sexual orientation (U.S. Department of Health and Human Services [USDHHS], 2001). The questions in the assessment boxes are intended to guide, not limit, the process of inquiry. Most of the questions are purposefully broad and open-ended. Special characteristics of particular communities most likely will generate additional or different questions, as well as different ways of categorizing the answers. Indeed, such departures from the assessment format presented in this book are encouraged as part of an in-depth and creative exploration of the community and its population.

Ordinarily assessment is preliminary to intervention, but community data cannot be collected all at once. It takes several months, even years, to know a whole community. Moreover, community assessment, like patient and family assessment, is an ongoing process and must be revised and updated regularly. Finally, all of the data compiled will not be of immediate use. These data, however, should be systematically recorded so that accurate information will be readily accessible when it is needed.

To formulate a healthy community agenda, information about health patterns, healthcare resources, and disease incidence and prevalence is not sufficient. All aspects of a community's health status are related to the contexts of community life in which they are manifested and addressed. High rates of cancer, for example, might be related to the presence of a nuclear energy plant and methods of waste disposal in one community, while in another they are linked to the age distribution of the population. Both age and exposure to toxic wastes are significant risk factors for cancer; however, the approach to addressing this situation in terms of advocacy, prevention, and interventions is significantly different for each community. In this example, a cultural assessment, using information about economic institutions and population distributions, enables the analysis of public health in relation to the community context and the development of an effective community health action plan.

Often, nurses who have worked in communities for a long time carry a community "data bank" around in their heads, containing information about residents, the environment, and community groups. Because they have internalized so much information about the community, it is not unusual for them to be unaware of how or why they decided on one course of action as opposed to another. While their decisions often are efficient and effective, they may be unable to muster the evidence required to justify a specific course of action. Community groups and boards that formulate policy and allocate resources are more likely to be persuaded by specific documentation than by the nurse's "intuition." The community nurse should have data readily available for purposes of discussion, planning, setting goals with professional and community groups, and for orienting new staff.

The degree to which community nurses succeed in building rapport and in accurately recording and reporting observations is directly related to the success of the community interventions. Like ethnographers, they become part of the situation they are trying to understand and manage and are, themselves, the data collection instruments (Sanday, 1979).

COMMUNITY CULTURAL ASSESSMENT PROCESS

When histories are conducted on individual patients, they are not random or haphazard processes. They consist of a systematic series of inquiries that help to order the findings about the patient so an accurate diagnosis can be made. There is an equally systematic way of examining communities to accomplish a logical progression of discovery. Many community health assessment tools begin with an appraisal of the actual and potential health problems experienced by community residents (Plescia, Koontz, & Laurent, 2001). The disadvantage of this strategy is that without knowing the context in which these problems are manifested, they are difficult to interpret and prioritize. Problems appear to occur in a vacuum instead of in relation to each other or in relation to other kinds of community problems. To determine whether they are, in fact, community health problems, it is necessary to learn about the wider community first, and then proceed to understanding its health (Butterfield, 1990, 2002).

GATHERING COMMUNITY DATA

A cultural assessment is derived from three basic sources:

- what can be observed directly about the community,

- what people say about the community, and

- what is written about the community in various documents, including historical sources, census reports, vital records, surveys, newspapers, and increasingly, data available on the World Wide Web.

There often is much confusion about the validity and reliability of various sources of data, and it is commonly suggested that direct observations are somehow less reliable because they are more "subjective." But even surveys and reports reflect the biases of both the subjects and the recorders. Survey data capture only the kind of information individuals and groups are willing to make public. Documents prepared by police de-

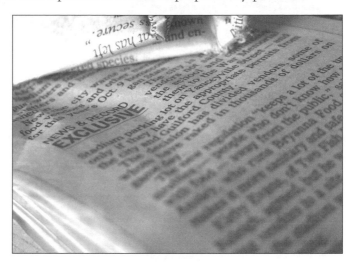

partments do not really tell us about the amount of criminal activity in a community. Rather, they tell us about the crimes that community residents choose to report or that police officers choose to record. Similarly, population statistics may grossly underestimate the size of a particular ethnic group if its members are legally undocumented. Thus, the source of data influences how the data are presented, interpreted, and used.

SELECTING THE SOURCE OF DATA

The superiority of some sources of information over others relates to the method of retrieval and to the question that is being asked. For example, if a community health nurse is exploring the nutritional status of schoolchildren, there are several approaches to gathering data:

- Ask children to complete a questionnaire on their 24-hour nutritional intake.

- Review the school menus over the past 3 months and evaluate the nutritional content of the meals.

- Rely on direct observations of eating behavior and food consumption by schoolchildren during mealtimes.

Each source of data has advantages and disadvantages. In the 24-hour nutritional intake questionnaire, the children may, consciously or unconsciously, report wholesome food consumption and neglect to mention the candy bar or potato chips purchased from

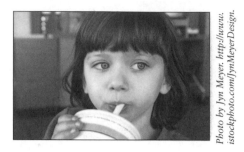

Photo by Jyn Meyer. http://www. istockphoto.com/JynMeyerDesign.

a vending machine. School menus provide reliable data on what was served but do not describe what was actually eaten. Direct observations, in this case, are probably the most revealing source of data, but very expensive to collect since the nurse cannot observe all the children at once. The most complete and easily obtained picture is derived from a combination of the three sources of data.

For some kinds of public health issues, direct observations may not be the best source of data. For example, formulating a 5-year plan for the provision of prenatal services in a designated population would rely heavily on census reports and data on migration patterns, economic changes, and birth and infant statistics over the past decade. In comparison, observations and interviews with childbearing women in prenatal clinics may be much less useful.

Different sources of data also permit the examination of both values and behaviors and the discrepancies that often exist between what people say and what people do. For example, community members may report they value good health and believe cigarette smoking is bad, yet observations reveal they continue to smoke. Teachers may instruct children in the principles of good nutrition in the classroom, but raise no objections to the installation of a candy vending machine in the school cafeteria. Identifying discrepancies and conflicts between what people say and what people do is essential for designing effective community health action plans.

DIRECT OBSERVATION

Participant observation in community life is a fundamental source of data and the hallmark of ethnographic methods. Much can be learned about the physical dimensions of the community and the lifestyles of its residents simply by walking or riding through designated areas. Street maps, obtained from local government offices or the chamber of commerce, are useful in guiding this preliminary observation of the community as a physical environment. Community observations should also include nights and weekends, and the four seasons. Community health practitioners who know the district only from 9 to 5, Monday through Friday, miss important information that may be vital in building community capacity. Attending public hearings, church services, and parent-teacher association meetings, as well as visiting shopping centers, school playgrounds, train stations, and movie theaters, reveal the culture of local life and group-held values.

INTERVIEWS OF COMMUNITY RESIDENTS

When using interviews and conversations as a source of data about the community, it is important to remember that each resident will provide a subjective description derived from his or her particular position in the community—the length of residence, occupation, neighborhood, age, and socioeconomic status. Therefore, it is not surprising that different members of the community will give very different—even conflicting—reports about the same community issue or event. One may claim a particular neighborhood is changing for the worse, while another may describe it as revitalized and an exciting place to live. The greater the variety of community residents surveyed, the more complete the picture of community culture will be. This includes not only those who are employed in or currently using the healthcare system, but also those who interact with the public on a routine basis and have a broad vision of the wider community (Bent, 2003): public officials, religious leaders, teachers, librarians, merchants, hairstylists, restaurant owners, bartenders, real estate brokers, bankers, journalists, or police officers.

Recently there has been considerable interest in *focus groups* as a means of collecting data that would help understand community health behavior and problems (Agar & MacDonald, 1995; Stevens, 1996; Swinney, Anson-Wonkka, Maki, & Corneau, 2001). Originating in market research companies, focus groups have become a frequently used method for gathering data in communities by public health and human services personnel. A focus group is composed of carefully selected individuals—usually 6 to 12—who engage in an exploratory meeting to discuss specific topics and offer opinions and experiences. The discussion is recorded and lasts about 1½ hours. Customarily, the groups are scheduled for at least one additional meeting after the participants have had an opportunity to review the first session, to assure that the topic is fully covered. In addition to providing useful data regarding a particular health problem, a focus group also serves to engage residents in community improvement. A community health nurse, for example, might use a focus group to examine the issue of expanding school-based health services. One focus group may consist of current or former students, teachers, members of the parent-teacher association, members of the school board, a pediatric nurse practitioner, and a pediatrician. Another focus group exploring this topic may consist solely of students and another solely of parents. Each group generates useful dialogue for determining the feasibility of a school-based health program. It also invests the participants in improving the health of school-age children and their families.

COMMUNITY DOCUMENTS

Two good documents to start learning about the community are the newspaper (including the small, advertisement-based papers) and the telephone directory. They are readily available and can provide a good introduction to the community culture. If the community does not have a newspaper of its own, the next most local newspaper often reveals the way in which the community is perceived regionally. The yellow pages of the telephone directory list hospitals, churches, recreational facilities, schools, day-care centers, physicians, lawyers, and other businesses and services available to residents. There also are many other formal sources of community data that already have been compiled. They can be found at the local library, chamber of commerce, government offices, department of education, police and fire departments, and parks and recreation offices. City or county planning commissions, if they exist, are particularly valuable sources of information, and sociodemographic data can be obtained from the most recent census (http://www.census.gov/), readily available on the Internet.

The same characteristics of data derived from interviews apply to data derived from documents. All documents, no matter how "objective," still reflect the perspective of the people and organizations that compiled them and the purpose for which they were to be used. Local newspapers, for example, will necessarily reflect the political and philosophical biases of the editors. Material assembled by the chamber of commerce will attempt to cast the community in a positive light in order to attract businesses. In comparison, data collected by the health department may be oriented more to community problems.

Unfortunately, documents that already have been prepared by various community organizations often are in units that are not coterminous with the designated study community. Information pertaining to children may have been compiled by school districts, data on communicable disease may have been compiled according to health districts, and data on public sanitation and safety may have been compiled according to fire and water districts or police districts. This is particularly true in more complex urban environments, where public institutions and offices have divided up the state, county, or city "pie" in different ways. Not only are these various "districts" not coterminous, they may cut across census tracks, as well as community boundaries.

RECORDING DATA

No matter which sources of data are used for the community assessment, it is always more helpful to report specific behavior and events than general impressions. In this respect, the information recorded in the community data bank is like the information recorded in a patient's chart, in which the nurse states exactly what is observed and heard. For instance, to report that "within the last year there were 22 incidents of assault and robbery in which the victim was 65 years or older, in comparison with 5 years earlier, when there were none," is more revealing than to say that "victimization of the elderly is a growing problem in this community." When an argument is based on actual data, it is more convincing. In this case, data citing the growing incidence of crimes against elder citizens helps to make a better argument for the allocation of funds to provide a transit service for the elderly or enhance the police protection for residents.

When recording interviews with community residents, their names and roles in the community should be noted. It is always more useful to record residents' own words and exact opinions than to give a generalized description. For example, reporting "Mr. Johnson, principal of Northside High School, would not support Representative Snyder in the next election because she opposed the introduction of sex education in the public school system" is more informative than reporting "community residents engaged in a lively discussion about sex education and local politics." In the first statement, the relationship among education, politics, and health is clear, not just from the perspective of *any* community resident, but from one who holds a pivotal position and works regularly in all three arenas. This more specific statement helps community health nurses understand current political issues, draw inferences about local sexual mores, and know who might support programs that address the issue of adolescent sexuality.

In public health, it is necessary to know not only *what* was said or written, but also *who* said or wrote it. This specificity requires recording the source of information as well as the information itself. If it is necessary to make estimates from statistical compilations intended for other purposes, the procedures and people used to obtain the estimate and the original purpose of the data should also be noted.

Finally, although the data bank must consist of accurate, specific information as opposed to just "impressions," a few comments about recording first impressions are in order. Impressions often change dramatically once one gets to know a community and its people. For example, Peace Corps workers have reported that on entering a third-world urban community, they were impressed with the crowded streets, the poorly clothed people, the disrepair of the housing, and the animals that seemed to wander freely, all giving the neighborhood an appearance of extreme poverty. After being in the country for several weeks, however, and exposed to other communities, they reclassified such communities as working-class. Although best clothes were reserved for church and work, and houses were modest, the families in these communities had access to resources, including live-stock, and were making strides toward social and economic improvement in a complex environment. Inferences always are subject to observer bias. It is important, nevertheless, to record first impressions and occasionally return to them. After living in a community for a while, one begins to take some of its characteristics for granted. First impressions serve as a reminder and actually help to retain a degree of objectivity. First impressions are also helpful in understanding the reactions of new-comers to the community.

> In public health, it is necessary to know not only *what* was said or written, but also *who* said or wrote it.

ANALYSIS OF DATA

The analysis of data collected during the community assessment is used to formulate a "healthy community agenda." Generally, analysis is the step that follows description. In community practice, however, data collection and analysis are processes. The first step in the analysis is to sort the data into useful categories. Not only is the community cultural assessment tool a useful reminder of the range of information needed to promote and sustain the health of the public, it also provides a way to classify information so that inferences can be drawn. This makes it possible to draw comparisons within the community or with state, regional, or national populations. It also allows for comparisons to be made regarding previous time periods, so current trends and the shifting patterns in community life can be understood.

For the purposes of analysis, there are four basic questions that should be asked of all the information obtained in the community assessment.

1. How do the data vary with time? For example, how do the number and quality of housing units compare with the previous 5 or 10 years?

2. How do the data compare with similar communities and with local, state, and national findings? For example, how does the proportion of residents over 65 compare with the proportion of those individuals at the state and national levels?

3. How are the findings in the various categories of the community cultural assessment related to findings in other categories? For example, how is education related to politics or economic factors?

4. What are the implications of the community cultural data for health and health-care? For example, what are the implications of a tourist-based economy for the health of community residents?

As mentioned earlier, these holistic, cultural assessments are not unlike the ethnographic methods used by anthropologists when they enter a culture unknown to them. Although the methods may be similar, the goals of the nurse and the anthropologist are quite different. The anthropologist is interested in explaining human behavior in all its cultural variations for the purpose of developing theories and knowledge about human nature. The community health nurse is interested in understanding human behavior and community culture for the purpose of building community capacity for better health. It is this goal—the assessment of cultural capital—that guides the process of assessment and analysis outlined in the following pages. The discussion associated with each set of questions is not intended to be an exhaustive presentation of all the possible inferences that could be drawn from each component of the community assessment. Rather, the discussion is intended to demonstrate how information about the community, which may appear at first to be unrelated to health and illness, is consequential in constructing a healthy community action plan.

> The community health nurse is interested in understanding human behavior and community culture for the purpose of building community capacity for better health.

THE COMMUNITY AS A PLACE IN TIME

The physical environment of a community, including its hills, rivers, buildings, street plan, and so forth, is among the most obvious aspects of community life. This physical environment is the setting for a population of citizens, whether the community is an urban neighborhood, a rural hamlet, or a coastal village. But the community is not only a population in *place;* it is also a population in *time* (Arensberg, 1954). Communities generally outlive their individual members. They have both a history and a future that influence what can be accomplished in the present. Successive generations, ranging from infants to seniors, reflect an orderly progression of the population through days, seasons and years that is just as much a part of community life as its rivers, roads, and buildings. Thus, in this first component of the community cultural assessment, the spatial and temporal aspects of community life will be examined.

SPATIAL DIMENSIONS OF COMMUNITY LIFE

People do not hang suspended in the atmosphere. They must occupy space and locate themselves on land or water. They both shape space and are shaped by it, and different communities occupy and use space and its contents in different ways. For example, many of the cities in the northeastern United States that were settled in the last century were built around a waterfall to power the textile or paper mills on which their economies were based. The typical settlement pattern in such communities consisted of worker houses built on flat ground, while the owners and high-level managers lived in more elegant accommodations on the hills (Arensberg, 1955). Examples of that type of settlement can be found in communities throughout New England. Midwestern agricultural communities, in comparison, were settled in family-dominated clusters of houses located in a more egalitarian manner, along roads leading to the town's "main street" commercial and service centers.

The spatial aspect of community life is a good place to initiate a community description, because it does not necessitate extensive interviews or informal discussions with residents.

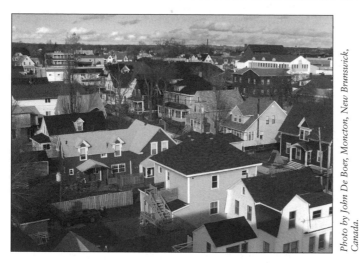

Photo by John De Boer, Moncton, New Brunswick, Canada.

With direct observation and reference to maps, much can be learned about the community, its health problems, and its resources. Community nurses working in remote areas of less technologically developed communities may find they will need to create their own maps indicating major topographical features and social institutions. Most communities, however, have fairly detailed maps that can be obtained from local planning departments or municipal or county offices.

Size and Boundaries

BOX #3.1

- **How large is the community in square miles?**

- **What are the boundaries of the community?**

Community nursing practice begins with knowing where the population or unit of service delivery begins and ends. It is therefore necessary to start by identifying the physical boundaries and the size, expressed in square miles, of the geographical territory to be served. Depending on the type of community, the size of its population, and the way in which it is organized, it could be geographically small, such as a city block, or it could encompass several rural counties. The physical size of the community in square miles will strongly influence the nature of community nursing practice. The nurse who is responsible for a district consisting of a few city blocks is likely to have daily face-to-face contact with many residents, while regular physical contact with residents scattered over many square miles may be supplemented by telephonic and electronic communication.

The kinds of boundaries that define a particular community also will influence the nature of community practice. For example, in settlements that are bounded by a river or a large highway, community practitioners may find the practice of public health delimited by those physical features. On the other hand, when the boundaries are more arbitrarily defined and one district blends imperceptibly into another, community health practice frequently will extend to families in adjoining blocks and will require significant collaboration with other health professionals in adjoining areas.

Regional Position

> **BOX #3.2**
>
> - **Is the community a service center for shopping, education, cultural events, healthcare, government activities, etc., or is it a satellite to a larger metropolitan center in which such services can be obtained?**
>
> - **Is there a commuting relationship between the community and other communities, e.g., work, kinship, leisure activities?**
>
> - **What is the distance, in time and miles, to the nearest urban center?**
>
> - **How does the community relate to the geopolitical units in which it is located? Is it a town, county, borough, village, or part of a municipality?**

The regional position of a community indicates how it is situated in relation to other communities—whether it is a satellite to a larger city or other municipality, or a center to which smaller communities are linked on a daily basis. The degree to which it is isolated from surrounding communities will influence the amount and nature of community health problems and the strategies and resources needed to resolve them. For example, in a community that is remote, the community nurse may need to emphasize self-help programs, such as first aid measures and health literacy. On the other hand, there are advantages to working in such communities, for kinship and neighbor networks can be mobilized more easily.

The regional position of communities and the amount of power and political influence such communities have are usually linked. Thus, the nurse working in a small, remote, satellite community may have a more difficult time effecting change or proposing new health policy than the nurse in the urban center where the most influential citizens live and the political constituencies are most powerful. This does not mean, however, that community health nurses in rural areas are powerless; it simply means different strategies must be deployed to accomplish community objectives, such as joining forces with other small communities in a regional effort.

The regional position of the community is also significant because many problems cannot be resolved at the local level. People may live in Community A, for example, but are getting sick where they work, in Community B. Individuals who travel daily from the suburbs to the city and back again to the suburbs are not only commuters, they also are potential carriers of health problems from one location to another. Thus, building the capacity of a community may require support from external sources unfamiliar with local level dynamics (Hill, 1986). The solutions to migrant worker health problems that affect many communities may require a collective petition for federal assistance. In addition to work ties, strong social ties often exist between members of communities that are geographically apart. For example, many Puerto Rican families living in New York travel back and forth regularly between Puerto Rico and New York, or they send their children to Puerto Rico during summer vacations to visit with grandparents. Knowledge of these ties is critical for understanding social and cultural institutions, assessing cultural capital, and building community capacity.

Geophysical and Climate Factors

BOX #3.3

- **What are the natural features of the environment that serve as an organizing force in the district/community (e.g., rivers, mountains, plains, coast)?**

- **What are the man-made features of the environment that serve as quasi-organic forces (e.g., superhighways, high-rise apartment complexes, industrial parks, bridges, tunnels)?**

- **What are the climatic conditions of the area (e.g., precipitation, winds, temperature range)?**

The topographical features of the community, such as mountains, rivers, or coastline, may be organizing forces in community life. Despite the extent to which humankind has reorganized the environment by building bridges, tunnels, and canals, cities continue to be affected by features of the natural environment. For example, four of the five boroughs of New York City are either islands or parts of islands. These features serve to define New York, especially the borough of Manhattan, as one in which growth must be vertical because there is no land for horizontal expansion. This feature is shared with urban island settlements, like Hong Kong. As in New York City, construction sites are common features of the landscape in Hong Kong where older buildings are being razed and replaced by newer, taller ones. In contrast, cities such as Los Angeles, Houston, and Dallas seem to sprawl indefinitely into their environments.

Topographical features impose various health threats on the community, such as mud slides, floods, forest fires, or earthquakes, and must be accounted for in a comprehensive healthcare plan for the community. In addition to the natural topography of communities, man-made physical features such as large, multilane highways, bridges, tunnels, and clusters of high-rise buildings or industrial parks serve as semi-organic forms that impact the health of communities and human activity. A superhighway, uniting several communities, makes it possible to centralize social and economic activities, expanding support for a healthy community agenda. At the same time, it may physically divide previously connected communities and impose several health hazards such as traffic accidents, air pollution, and harmful noise levels.

Land Use

- **Outline the functional designations of land in the community. What areas are specified for residential, recreational, commercial, industrial, agricultural, official, and spiritual or religious use?**

- **What are the patterns of land use by the population? Which areas are open to all? Which areas are open to specific members of the population, such as the old, young, men, women, or certain ethnic groups?**

Communities create various kinds of boundaries. Some have settlement patterns where sections of the community are designated for a special function, such as residential, commercial, industrial, governmental, spiritual, or recreational. Other communities exist, however, where residents sleep, eat, work, play, and worship all within the range of a few blocks, and there is no geographical separation of these various human activities. The designation of different locations for different functions of daily living generates patterns of assemblage and dispersal of community residents. Gathering points such as commercial centers or industrial complexes may bring community members together for certain periods of the day or week, while scattered residences take them in separate directions for the remainder of the time.

One of the decisions community health nurses may be called upon to make is how to affect the greatest number of people. Without knowledge about the way in which members of the population use space, it is difficult to make such decisions. It is thus important to identify areas of assemblage where many of the residents can conveniently be reached. For example, in some communities, the most efficient way to reach larger numbers of adults might be through industry where they are employed. However, in places such as agricultural-based communities, where adults work in highly dispersed patterns, weekly meetings of the local farmers association may be the best place to meet adult residents. One resourceful community health nurse discovered elders could be reached at a local restaurant where they gathered to have breakfast each day. The nurse not only monitored the health of this subpopulation, but also engaged this network of elder clients in community development.

Other communities may be organized according to the special characteristics of the residents, such as ethnicity ("Little Italy" or "China Town"), or by class (the "ghettos" or the "Peacock Hills"), or even by occupation, such as enclaves of artists and musicians or university faculty. Many U.S. communities have been and continue to be characterized by segregation (Azevedo-Garcia, Lochner, Osypuk, & Subramanian, 2003)—one of the principal reasons for the movement to desegregate school districts, a movement that gripped this country during much of the latter part of the 20th century (Lucas, 1986). These cultural specifications of territory within communities highlight health disparities. Specific groups may informally designate a particular area of the community as their own "turf" and create boundaries that are not visible to the outsider, but are well-known and well-respected by local residents.

When attention is not paid to questions of access in a community (i.e., who may go where), the health of a community is often compromised. One such case was a lead-screening program held at a fast-food restaurant on a Saturday. A favorite gathering spot for young families on the weekend, the restaurant was considered an ideal site for reaching preschool-age children. Indeed, in terms of the number of children screened, it was extremely successful. In terms of reaching the population most at risk, however, the program failed. No one had taken into consideration that the lower income families in which children were most likely to have lead exposure could not afford to bring their children to the fast food restaurant. A better understanding of the distribution of people in the community and differential access to space could easily have averted the problem and saved the necessary expense of an additional program.

Housing

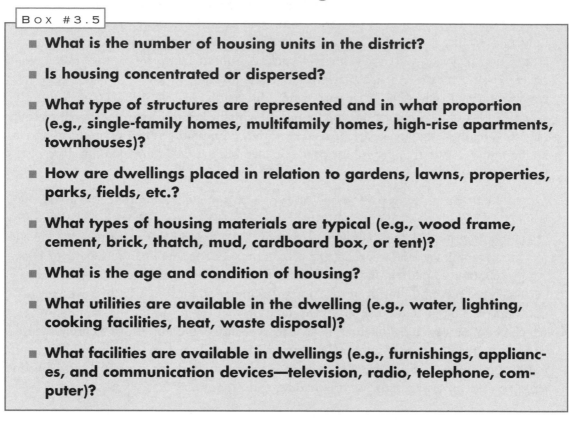

BOX #3.5

- **What is the number of housing units in the district?**

- **Is housing concentrated or dispersed?**

- **What type of structures are represented and in what proportion (e.g., single-family homes, multifamily homes, high-rise apartments, townhouses)?**

- **How are dwellings placed in relation to gardens, lawns, properties, parks, fields, etc.?**

- **What types of housing materials are typical (e.g., wood frame, cement, brick, thatch, mud, cardboard box, or tent)?**

- **What is the age and condition of housing?**

- **What utilities are available in the dwelling (e.g., water, lighting, cooking facilities, heat, waste disposal)?**

- **What facilities are available in dwellings (e.g., furnishings, appliances, and communication devices—television, radio, telephone, computer)?**

Housing plays an important role in providing a safe, healthy, comfortable, and aesthetically pleasing context for individual and family growth. In addition to providing shelter for a population, it is directly related to the quality of family relationships and to both the psychological and physical dimensions of health. The type of construction and the placement of housing units in relation to each other and to community gathering points influence the way in which residents interact. Apartment buildings in which there is a common courtyard, swimming pool, or laundry area, for example, are likely to foster a greater "community spirit" among residents of the building than a high-rise, dormitory-like building where one rarely sees the person who lives in the apartment next door. Many cities, such as Chicago, are replacing high-rise dwellings with three-story, townhouse-type housing for this reason.

Access to a piece of land for gardens or recreation is another important feature of housing. Many innovative urban residents have transformed vacant lots into vegetable gardens, subdivided and tended by apartment dwellers. In addition to solving the aesthetic and safety problems that accompany vacant lots, such gardens provide city residents with the opportunity to produce, preserve, and perhaps even sell fresh food. Finally, such community gardens often become a focal point for community activity, such as outdoor markets, thus enhancing relationships among residents.

Housing must be examined in relation to the characteristics of the people residing in the community. It may be very difficult for a specific ethnic group living in adobe, single-story homes with a detached kitchen to adjust to the high-rise housing of urban centers. Housing units that were constructed for one population group, such as young families, may be inconvenient for elders who may require elevators, wheelchair ramps, or different kinds of lighting. Much of modern housing is electricity-dependent and subject to energy crises in summer or winter months, creating a potentially serious problem for elder residents. Finally, abandoned housing has generated a widespread environmental safety problem. Condemned buildings may attract urban squatters, illicit drug users, homeless people, and even neighborhood children looking for a place to play.

Transportation and Communication

> **Box #3.6**
>
> - **What are the patterns of spatial movement within and between residences, workplaces, commercial centers, schools, etc.?**
>
> - **Outline the transportation system and communication network, including major arteries, available routes, and public and private transportation (e.g., bus lines, subway, taxi, trains, air travel, water routes).**
>
> - **What forms of transportation link the community with the nearest urban centers?**
>
> - **What forms of communication exist within the community and connect it to other communities (e.g., newspapers, radio stations, television stations)?**

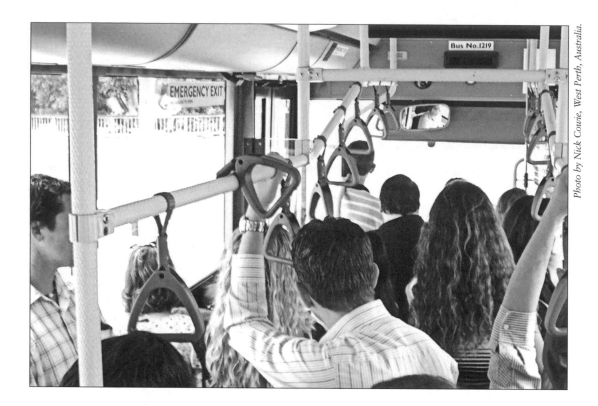

Photo by Nick Cowie, West Perth, Australia.

The designation of different zones for different community functions and events requires a transportation system to move the population from one activity to another. In addition to knowing about the way land is used in the community, it is also necessary to understand the network of roads, waterways, and other public transportation. An example of what can happen when this aspect of community life is not considered is provided by a case in which a hospital in a large city decided to close its pediatric clinic. Even before it was phased out, health planners in the geographically nearest hospital began to plan for the influx of families they assumed would be drawn from the closed service. The planners, however, did not account for the fact that even though it was the closest hospital by distance, the journey to the new clinic required a transfer from one bus line to another. Most patients found it more convenient to go to another clinic that was actually farther away, but could be reached on one bus line, without the hassle of transfer.

The communication system is perhaps the community practitioner's most important capacity-building tool. Radio stations and newspapers link individuals and groups, both within and outside the community for health education, disaster preparedness, and public participation. In one city, ethnic disparities in health were linked to language differences and health literacy. One suggestion was to send out a health newsletter that would be translated and disseminated to all residents in the community. However, an analysis of the communication networks suggested it would be more efficient to send health information to the many well-read ethnic newspapers that already existed in this multicultural community. Health editors of local newspapers and hosts of local television health programs are important resources for disseminating correct information about health and for assuring the participation of community residents in health issues. Some nurses have even initiated their own health columns and television and radio programs in an attempt to reach the public (Mason, 2000).

Mental Maps

BOX #3.7

- **What sections are distinguished by the residents themselves, and what names or nicknames are applied to them?**

- **What are the psychological barriers that exist in the community? What areas of the community are frequently avoided or feared by residents, and what areas are seen as safe?**

- **Are there parts of the community that are designated as sacred, or historical areas such as ancient burial grounds, memorial parks, etc.?**

Some individuals depict a view of the United States from a New Yorker's perspective, which, looking west, includes first New Jersey and then the West Coast with nothing in between except Chicago. The person living in Missouri, Montana, or Alabama would have, of course, a very different, but perhaps equally distorted, mental image of the United States. Residents also may have a view of their community that is not congruent with the way the community practitioner sees it. Social scientists have, for several years, used "mental maps" (drawings done by residents of their community) to discover the interface of the psychological topography with the physical topography. In doing so, they have identified invisible "peaks" of psychic stress, where residents are afraid to walk, and "valleys" of safety, where they feel comfortable and unafraid.

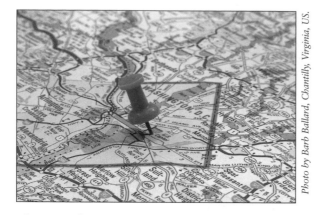

Photo by Barb Ballard, Chantilly, Virginia, US.

The names and nicknames applied to certain neighborhoods and sections of the community also tell much about how various neighborhoods are viewed. It is not unusual, for instance, for neighborhoods that have undergone extensive gentrification to have two names: one that is used by the residents who were born and grew up in the neighborhood and another that is used by the wealthier newcomers. This use of two names to describe the same place is telling. It mirrors the social and economic differences between the two types of residents and indicates not only how various residents perceive themselves, but also about the relations between them. It alerts community health nurses that there might be a need to use a different strategy with each category of resident. As with the "turf" aspects described earlier, sacred areas, areas of fear or safety, and other psychological features are superimposed on the physical features. They often are not demarcated and go unnoticed by the newcomer to the community. Sensitivity to "mental maps" is important, however, for understanding the perception people have of their environments.

MANAGING SPATIAL DATA

Community practice nurses should have at their disposal several maps or charts. These can include: (a) a map that outlines the major topographical features of the community (mountain ranges, hills, rivers, lakes and ponds, seashore, etc.); (b) a map that designates the regional position of the district/community and urban centers and outlines the transportation system in and out; and (c) a map that denotes settlement patterns, streets, highways, residential areas, commercial and other functional areas, and major institutions such as schools, churches, commercial centers, and official buildings. These will provide the backdrop of the aspects of community life that are relevant to the practice of public health. This includes routine movement of the population within the community, public gathering places, ethnic enclaves, tracts of poor housing, congested streets, high crime areas, and environmental hazard areas (flooding, forest fires, and hurricanes). Locations of health problems, such as animal and insect pests, epidemics, polluted water, traffic accidents, and high crime areas can then be denoted against this environmental backdrop for purposes of analysis and planning. Such maps should be part of the arsenal of community practice nurses and treated as "working documents" to which new information can always be added.

TEMPORAL DIMENSIONS OF COMMUNITY LIFE

Each community has its own cycle of activities and behavior. These temporal factors are especially important in community health practice, because timing is an essential component when planning community interventions. If immunization programs are offered at a time when they are inaccessible to community residents, the participation rate will be low. Similarly, political action related to health may be reserved for election time, when an issue is most likely to get support from a political candidate and have the greatest impact. While all nurses are concerned with time and timing, these concepts are particularly important in community practice, where the timing of interventions must be culturally appropriate to succeed. For this reason, a cultural assessment of the temporal aspects of community life should begin with an overview of its history.

Community History

BOX #3.8

- **When was the community first settled and what were the circumstances surrounding the settlement?**

- **What have been the patterns of population growth in the community since it was first settled, including waves of migration?**

- **What have been the milestone events in the history of the community, including both natural and man-made events (e.g., economic changes; wars; opening of new roads, railroads, or bridges; disasters)?**

- **What are the major physical alterations that have occurred and when?**

- **What changes in settlement patterns have taken place throughout the history of the community (e.g., a shift of the commercial center from "downtown" to suburban shopping centers)?**

- **What have been the major economic trends in the community?**

- **What have been the major political trends in the community?**

The community of today is largely a result of its history, because specific events and trends have worked to shape the place and its people. Knowledge of the history of the community is important for tracing and interpreting patterns of health problems over time and predicting those that will occur in the future (Dressler, 1991). Understanding the local history can help the nurse develop a practice that is predictive and yet blends with community traditions (Munhall, 1992).

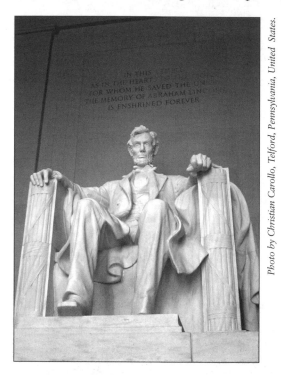

Photo by Christian Carollo, Telford, Pennsylvania, United States.

Historical details of the community are not as important as general knowledge of what has made the community what it is. There may already be a history written about the community, either because it has a particularly interesting history or because it was done as part of a community event. If there is no history available in the library or official archives of the municipality or county, there are other sources of history ordinarily available, such as interviews with older residents, old newspapers and public records, census reports, school records, directories, deeds, old maps, and church records.

Cyclical Population Movement

BOX #3.9

■ **What patterns of population movement characterize the community on a daily, weekly, seasonal, or annual basis?**

■ **How do these vary for the subpopulations within the community (e.g., by age, sex, ethnicity, class, occupation)?**

To provide efficient, accessible, and appropriate health services, it is very important to know the daily, weekly, seasonal, and annual changes in the population. The movement of people from one place to another generally takes place with a degree of regularity and needs to be accommodated in assuring the health and safety of community residents. For example, if the safety of children coming and going to school has been identified as a community health priority, it will be necessary to know when automobile traffic is heaviest and when children are most at risk.

Seasonal changes in the population are equally significant and often the cause of shifts in population: for example, the presence of migrant workers during the summer months or the dramatic shifts in the population of university towns when thousands of students arrive in the fall and depart in the spring. These seasonal fluctuations in population size have a profound effect on the type and quantity of health problems that must be identified and resolved within the resources of the community. Seasonal changes also significantly affect the economic statistics of the community, from which many state and federal aid programs derive formulas for aid. Resort areas experience similar fluctuations. The summer population of tourists in small, ocean resort towns far exceeds that in the winter, presenting challenges for creating a safe, healthy community all year long. Just the opposite occurs in the South, where a typically elder population is greatest in the winter. Multi-annual population shifts are evident in some communities. In Washington, DC, for example, national elections bring about changes in the population every two years. As some members of Congress and their aides and families move out, a new set of government officials and personnel move in. Priorities for community practitioners working in places that experience dramatic seasonal fluctuations might include the development of an orientation program for new residents to the community and its health.

Economic Cycles

BOX #3.10

- **What are the changes in the patterns of work in the community (e.g., regular periods of unemployment, cycles of productivity, seasonal occupational changes)?**

- **Are there periodic changes in income, expenditures, or cash flow?**

This category of the community assessment includes temporal variations in the local economic structure, including cyclical variations in productivity, employment, occupation, income, and expenditures. The influence of seasonal variation in the local economy on health and healthcare is apparent in agricultural communities. In countries that engage in the production of sugar cane, for example, hundreds of workers are employed during a 6-month period, both in the field to cut the cane and in the factory to process it into sugar. During this time, cash is in highest circulation and people have the resources to pay off their debts and make new purchases. It is also the time when utilization of healthcare services increases dramatically. There are two reasons for this: One is that working in the cane fields and factories increases the incidence of accidents; the second is that there is more money in circulation to take care of deferred health problems. In the *Healthy People 2010* document, agriculture is one of the industries with the highest rate of traumatic deaths. The construction industry also has a high rate of traumatic death; both are highly seasonal industries (USDHHS, 2001).

In community health, timing is a large part of the success of any healthy community agenda. A community's health from January to July may be quite different from August to September. Each season presents both challenges and opportunities for building community capacity.

Psychological Cycles

BOX #3.11

- **What are the psychological cycles of the community?**

- **What are the periods of euphoria and dysphoria?**

- **What are the periods of festivities and holidays?**

- **When do the opportunities for personal life, leisure, and recreation occur?**

- **Are periods of widespread melancholy present in the community (e.g., seasonal affective disorder)?**

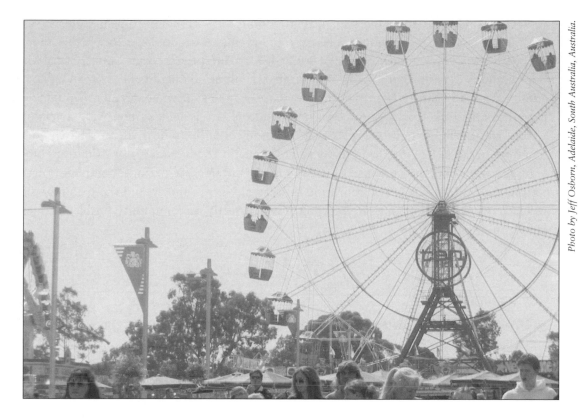

Photo by Jeff Osborn, Adelaide, South Australia, Australia.

Communities have periodic cycles when either psychological elevation or depression is generalized throughout the population. In most American communities, holidays and other times of ceremonial activity are seen as periods when there is a great deal of anticipation and enthusiasm, with opportunities to be with family and renew old friendships. Often such a "euphoric" season is followed by a more depressed one in which the excitement of the holidays is over, work has resumed, bills must be paid, and weather keeps people indoors and isolated from friends and recreational activity. The first warm days then bring a return of the euphoria, with the anticipation of spring and summer and the resumption of social interaction. Many nurses and physicians working in community mental health centers recognize these cyclical fluctuations in community mood and anticipate seasonal patterns of utilization.

Nurses working in student health centers report similar patterns. Each semester begins with the excitement of new classes and new friends. Then as the semester wears on, students are faced with assignments, tests, and papers to be completed, and a fairly predictable midterm depression sets in. At that point, it is common to hear students say they cannot wait for the semester to be over and even express doubt as to whether they will be able to complete their course of study. It is during these periods of dysphoria when absenteeism is most likely to occur, comparatively minor complaints take on an enhanced significance, and visits to health services increase. At the same time, faculty members feel an additional stress—perhaps in response to students—creating a system-wide dysphoria. In contrast, during periods of euphoria, it is not uncommon to hear students say, "I don't have time to get sick; I'm getting ready to go home for the holidays," or "I'm not going to miss homecoming just because I have the flu." During these periods, complaints are minimized and health services utilization decreases. Nurses understand these community level variations in mood and can interpret them correctly as community problems amenable to community solutions.

Cyclical Crises

BOX #3.12

- **What are the recurring and sporadic crises that occur in the community?**

- **What has been the response of the community?**

Practically all communities have crises that recur on a fairly predictable schedule. Spring flooding, annual flu epidemics, seasonal drownings, and summer fires are common examples of critical events that take place more or less regularly. Drowning, the second leading cause of injury-related death in children and adolescents, is clearly a seasonal event (USDHHS, 2001). Because seasonal events are relatively predictable, community health nurses can institute action that may or may not prevent events, but minimally will avert the crises that accompany them. For example, community nurses practicing in a remote mountainous community reported bringing pregnant women across the river each year before the rainy season, when the normally shallow and easily fordable river began to swell. This is another example of community practice nurses working in the future, anticipating problems, and finding ways to ameliorate them or soften their impact. If most drownings occur during the summer months, a prevention program on water safety and first aid should be presented just before children leave school for their summer vacations, when the information will have the most impact. A major responsibility of community health nurses working in the southeast United States is to assure residents are properly educated and prepared for a hurricane: that they have an adequate supply of food and know how to treat water so it is potable. They also must work with other agencies in the community to coordinate appropriate evacuation procedures and inform residents where to go for shelter and when they must leave their homes.

In addition to the seasonal crises that occur with a fair degree of regularity, there are others that occur infrequently or simply have the potential for occurring. Fires, tornadoes, tsunamis, earthquakes, major epidemics, mining disasters, nuclear disasters, and now, of course, terrorist attacks, all require advance action. The goal is to develop and maintain the community's capacity for readiness to reduce the impact by having a plan in place. This does not mean community health nurses are totally responsible for the management of crises and disasters. It does mean, however, the potential for such crises should be identified in a community assessment and a plan should be in place to handle such events, working with other health and human service professionals, including sanitation and safety engineers, police, communications networks, and rescue teams.

MANAGING TIME-SPECIFIC DATA

The time-specific aspects of community life should be recorded on a series of schedules and calendars representing daily, weekly, and seasonal variations in community activity. It is possible that each subgroup within a community will have a different schedule and cycle of activities, and thus separate records are necessary for special groups. Some of these data can be collected from calendars prepared by schools, churches, health agencies, industries, recreational facilities, and planning agencies. Community celebrations and holidays should be recorded on community calendars, along with major religious festivals, school vacations and events, ethnic celebrations, historical occasions, etc. Psychological euphoric and dysphoric cycles also are recorded on these calendars, as are seasonal shifts in economic activity. The goal is to be as comprehensive as possible, and the calendars, like the maps of topographical features and settlement patterns, are "working documents," always being revised and updated. A good calendar probably will not look very tidy, but will provide a useful guide to the activity of community life.

The value of knowing the time-specific dimensions of community life cannot be overestimated. An example of this occurred in a family planning project in a rural Caribbean community. The project was well-designed from a technical standpoint. To bring family planning education to rural communities, a van had been fully equipped with its own electric generator, a film projector, and a full assemblage of family planning materials. Family planning educators were selected and trained and were scheduled to visit several communities each week. The presentations were usually scheduled for evenings on a weeknight and ordinarily were filled to capacity. Unfortunately, those who attended were either children, men, or older women. All the women of childbearing age were home looking after their small children. While it is certainly advantageous for all community residents to be exposed to the concept of family planning, particularly young men and adolescents of both sexes, the target population for whom the program was intended was not there. The program planners had neglected to take into consideration that in rural Caribbean communities, men are nighttime gatherers while women are daytime gatherers. Had the program been held on Sunday at various churches in the community, in the marketplace on Saturday, or at rural clinics on a weekday, it is likely more women of childbearing age would have been reached directly.

The Total Population

BOX #3.13

- **What is the size of the population of the community?**

- **What is the density of the population (i.e., people per square mile)?**

- **What is the distribution of the population between urban and rural areas?**

- **What are the patterns of population change due to migration and natural increase (births and deaths)?**

The second component of a community cultural assessment is an examination of the culture's actors—its population. The number of people in a community and their attributes will influence the capacity of a community to create a healthy future. The population can be examined as a whole in terms of its size, growth, and distribution. It also can be examined in terms of the biocultural and socioeconomic characteristics of its members. These characteristics tell us much about the kinds of health problems that can be anticipated; they also provide information about the strengths of the population and how a healthy community agenda can be facilitated.

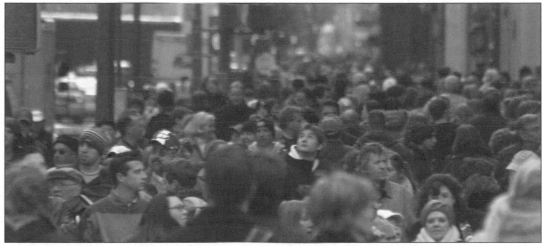

Photo by Lior Angel, Tel Aviv, Israel.

POPULATION SIZE, DENSITY, AND DISTRIBUTION

An assessment of the population begins with the knowledge of how many people reside in the community. Is the community practitioner responsible for the health of a public consisting of 1,000, 5,000, or 20,000 people? The number of residents a single community health nurse can effectively manage depends greatly on the density of the population. Rural localities have been highlighted in *Healthy People 2010* as one of the six factors accounting for the nation's health disparities. Defined as communities with fewer than 2,500 residents, rural residents comprise 25% of the American population and have health-related needs that are unique to rural conditions and lifestyle (USDHHS, 2001). Some communities have both urban and rural sections, or areas of high and low density. Constructing a healthy community agenda requires knowing how the population is distributed.

In addition to current size and density, the community health nurse must be able to anticipate public health problems that will accompany population changes. This begins with an accounting of population trends over the past several years, including patterns of migration—both into and away from the community—and natural increases or decreases, determined by birth and death rates (Norman, Boyle, & Rees, 2004; Urrutia-Rojas & Aday, 1991).

Temporary Subpopulations

BOX #3.14

- **Are there temporary subpopulations that live within the community?**

Some communities have special groups such as the military, summer residents, students, migrant workers, or other groups who may currently *reside* in the community but are not *from* the community. In some instances, such groups may strain community resources, compromising community capacity for health. On the other hand, they may contribute to the economy of the community and have positive attributes that enhance the cultural capital of the community. In any case, the presence of these groups must be accounted for in ensuring the future health of the community. This includes identifying their numbers, major characteristics, roles within the community, prevailing health problems, and the resources they can offer to community health.

Biological Composition: Age and Sex

BOX #3.15

- **What is the median age of the population?**

- **What percentage of the population is under age 15, 15-19, 20-34, 35-49, 50-64, and 65 and over?**

- **What is the dependency ratio of the population?**

- **What is the sex composition of the population?**

- **What is the sex ratio of the population?**

- **What is the age/sex quotient of the population?**

When providing direct nursing care to individual patients, it is necessary to know their biological characteristics in order to make accurate nursing diagnoses and formulate appropriate care plans. The same principle holds true when providing care to an entire community. The age and sex distribution of a population tells us much about the kinds of health problems the population is likely to experience now and in the future. Age and sex are, perhaps, the most fundamental of the biological characteristics, because so many community health problems are linked to changes in developmental cycles and to sex.

The aging of populations throughout the country has mandated a shift in emphasis from child health and infectious disease to management of the chronically ill and elder community residents. The first goal of *Healthy People 2010*, increasing the quality and years of healthy life, for "graying" communities, will require different orientations, knowledge, and ways of organizing for community health (Craig, 1994; Schultz & Magilvy, 1988). The second—eliminating health disparities—also is a challenge in aging communities, often composed mostly of women (USDHHS, 2001).

In statistical compilations, the age of a population is presented as the percentage of the population that falls into the various categories identified above. These categories, however, may be more or less useful depending on the nature of the community. For example, if community health nurses are working in a setting that has a very large proportion of elderly residents, the "over 65" group might be subdivided into the "young elderly" of 65 to 74, the "mid-elderly" of 75 to 84, and the "frail elderly" of 85 and over. At the same time, two of the adult categories might be collapsed into one large group from 35 to 64, simply because the community doesn't have large numbers of individuals in those particular age groups. In other words, for purposes of public health, the categories should be refined in a way that makes most sense and is most useful for the particular community. The proportion of the population that is under 20 and over 65 is computed as the dependency ratio, meaning it is the part of the total population that is considered to be economically and socially dependent on the rest of the population. It is also the proportion of the population that is most vulnerable in terms of health and that uses the greatest proportion of health services. It is therefore a significant figure for public health consideration.

Men and women differ in the kinds of health problems they experience and the manner and frequency with which they use health services. While acknowledging some sex-specific health problems are biologically based, *Healthy People 2010* highlights sex as one of the six categories in which health disparities must be addressed. Why women's life expectancy exceeds that of men by six years, and what accounts for the differing occurrence of depression, injury, and Alzheimer's disease between men and women, are probably not solely biologically based (USDHHS, 2001). An accounting of sex and gender in the community thus permits the public health nurse to make predictions about both potential and prevailing health problems, and to plan the resources required to deal with them. As the sex that bears children and generally lives longer, women use more health services than men. Furthermore, health problems that were once attributable primarily to men, such as cardiovascular disease, now are recognized with increasing frequency among women (Sorlie, Backlund, & Keller, 1995).

A high sex ratio, that is, a predominance of either men or women, often is typical of immigrant groups, migrant work camps, or military communities. Obviously, communities where men predominate would have less need for gynecological, prenatal, or pediatric services. On the other hand, the decreased emphasis on women's health in such communities would require greater vigilance on the part of the nurse to assure the health needs of women are addressed.

Once the age and sex composition of the community has been determined, it is useful to cross tabulate these two factors in order to know the sex ratio within each age category. This greater refinement of the age and sex data permits even more predictability as each age group moves to the next developmental stage. For example, it is usually assumed the 65 and older category is predominantly female, but a closer investigation of the community may reveal military service and migration have left one community lacking in males in one age group and increasing their proportion in another. In New York's Chinatown, for example, the elderly population has been, for several years, predominantly male, reflecting the wave of Chinese immigrant men who came to the United States in the first half of the 20th century as laborers. As each age group moves through its next developmental sequence, its sex composition will have an impact on the health of the community and the necessary health services.

Racial and Ethnic Groups

BOX #3.16

- **List the various ethnic groups found in the community.**

- **Calculate each ethnic group's percentage of the total population.**

- **List the various racial groups in the community.**

- **Calculate each racial group's percentage of the total population.**

- **What percentage of the population identifies itself as multiracial?**

- **How homogeneous or diverse are the various racial and ethnic groups?**

Race and ethnicity are also highlighted by *Healthy People 2010* as being linked to health disparities in the United States. Ethnicity and race are two distinct categories that sometimes overlap but often are incorrectly collapsed into one. Ethnicity is the complex of cultural traits that characterize a group of people based on common ancestry, including language, religion, diet, child-rearing practices, gender roles, and family composition and dynamics. Race, on the other hand, is a more controversial concept (Harrison, 1998; Montague, 1997; Wolf, 1994). While commonly thought of as a biological attribute, based on a person's phenotype and genotype, contemporary social science conceptualizes race as a socially constructed category. In the United States, for example, a person whose appearance (or phenotype) is "white" is considered "black" if his mother happens to be African American. "Hispanic" is a common racial category on health and census surveys. This category implies, incorrectly, that people of Spanish origin are a separate racial group from white or black. Neither race nor ethnicity can be determined from an individual's phenotype or genotype. Since census reports and health surveys, however, often use racial categories that group people according to white, black or Hispanic, it is important to have a basic understanding of current conceptions of race.

Contemporary population geneticists group people into "demes," or breeding groups, that are geographically clustered (Holloway, 2003; Templeton, 1998). The homogeneity of a population, both in genotypic and phenotypic terms, is dependent on the proximity of different breeding groups as well as the geographic mobility of the group through migration. Large populations, such as the Chinese, that are separated from other large populations, such as Europeans, often have significant phenotypic differences from each other. These populations have been referred to in racial terms—"mongoloid" and "caucasoid," respectively. Populations located at the intersection of the two large groups are known as clinal populations. Members of *clinal* populations, such as those of western Asia, are likely to share the phenotypic and genotypic features of the two larger, more homogeneous groups (Holloway, 2003).

Thus, the Chinese, on average, share phenotypic and genotypic characteristics that distinguish them from European populations. Intervening groups (Afghanis, Nepalese, Tibetans, and some Russian populations, for example) are clinal populations relative to the Chinese and European. Of course, the distribution of genotypical and phenotypical characteristics is affected by geography, (i.e., high mountain ranges), social intercourse (i.e., trade), and cultural and political events (i.e., marriage rules and war) that would inhibit or promote contact between two groups. In most cases, referring to any individual or group using racial terms—negroid, mongoloid, caucasoid—is not very useful, since most of the world's population doesn't fit into these tidy categories and, if globalization continues at its current rate, it will be even less so. Because, however, the concept of race continues to be used in public surveys as a means of identifying populations at risk, its usage in this text will reflect common cultural usage, without assigning biological attributes.

With the geographical clustering of populations, it is not uncommon for specific health problems to have a genetic origin and thus appear with greater frequency in some groups than in others. It is well-known, for example, that sickle-cell anemia is found more often in the African-American populations, Tay-Sachs disease in some Jewish groups, skin cancer in those of northern European ancestry, and diabetes in some American Indian groups. Certain groups also have inherited resistance to specific diseases. Cancer, for instance, is comparatively low in American Indian populations (Brownson, Patrick, & Davis, 1993). Thus, at the community level, race and ethnicity can inform the identification of risk for problems likely to require public health action such as screening and health education.

Many health problems that are *correlated* with ethnicity and race are not *caused* by an inherited predisposition, but rather are associated with social position, socioeconomic status, or conditions of employment of particular groups or subgroups (Boone, 1989; Krieger, Chen, Waterman, Rekpopf, & Subramanian, 2005; Singh & Yu, 1995; Sorlie, Backlund, & Keller, 1995). The combination of biological and social factors can result in variable health status. The higher rate of hypertension in some African-American and other groups has been related to the stress associated with a lifetime of discrimination (Bhui et al., 2005; Dressler, Grell, & Viteri, 1995; Grim & Wilson, 1993; Guralnik & Leveille, 1997).

Prejudice and discrimination have not been confined to racial groups, as the history of the Irish and Eastern European Jews in 19th- and 20th-century America attests. In cases where discrimination has been legally sanctioned, such as African-American populations until the 1950s, the quality and quantity of prejudice has been particularly horrific. Well into the 20th century, for example, blacks were prohibited by law from patronizing many restaurants, hotels, healthcare facilities, educational institutions, and so on. These qualitative and quantitative disparities must be acknowledged to appreciate the vast differences that characterized various ethnic or racial groups over time (Carlson & Chamberlain, 2004; Mullings, 1978).

Race and ethnicity can have a profound influence on the health and sustainability of communities (Meleis, Lipson, & Paul, 1992). They can be the source of community conflict, isolation, uneven distribution of resources, poor health, and ultimately health disparities. On the other hand, as cultural capital, they may be a source of strength and richness in mobilizing and uniting communities. The racial and ethnic mix of a community is simply another population variable that must be accounted for in engaging in community health action, and may pale in comparison to other impediments to healthy community relations (Eberhardt & Pamuk, 2004; Higgs, Boyne, & Murphy, 2001; Melnyk, 1988).

Occupation, Income and Education Level

BOX #3.17

- **What is the per capita income in the community?**
- **What is the mean and median family income and household income?**
- **What is the percentage of the population with incomes below poverty level?**
- **What is the percentage of the population receiving public assistance?**
- **What is the unemployment rate?**
- **What is the percentage of women in the workforce?**
- **What is the percentage of men in the workforce?**
- **What are the major occupational categories comprising the population (professionals, technical workers, managers, officials, proprietors, crafts-men, artisans, operatives, farmers, laborers, domestic workers, etc.)?**
- **What percentage of the population over age 25 has completed high school?**
- **What percentage of the population over age 25 has completed college?**

Income and occupation influence many aspects of health and healthcare. There is no question that populations with high rates of unemployment, poverty, and public assistance will generate different health problems (Abraham, 1993; Rodwin & Neuberg, 2005). Generally, the problems in poorer communities are more complex, because the resources to resolve them are more difficult to obtain. Inequality in income is another of the six areas highlighted in the *Healthy People 2010* document as underlying health disparities. Together with inequality in education, poverty characterizes those groups that suffer the worst health status (USDHHS, 2001).

In assessing the occupation and income of a population, it is important to remember that indicators such as average income per household must be evaluated within the local economic context. An average family income of $40,000 per year may be more than sufficient to meet the household needs of families living in the rural Midwest United States, but totally inadequate for a similar family residing in Southern California or Boston, MA. Differences in economic profile are associated with other differences, such as age distribution or ethnicity. When analyzing the income of a population, the community health nurse must compare it with similar populations in the region and nationally.

In addition to knowing the income level, knowing the occupational composition of the population provides information about the kinds of potential health problems that prevail in the community. For example, workers in mining and textile manufacturing are at risk for respiratory problems, and office workers are at risk for carpal tunnel syndrome. Just as with age, sex, race, and ethnicity, occupation allows us both to predict and to prevent health problems in a population (Landrigan, 1992).

The proportion of adult females in the workforce is equally revealing. First, it suggests there is a need to examine the effects of employment and occupation on women's health, including fertility. Second, it requires a look at the caregiving function of families. The women's movement has done much to enhance the status of women, but the increasing numbers of women in the workforce over the past three decades have left many communities without their traditional caregivers. Communities already have responded to this with the establishment of community day-care centers, not only for preschoolers but also for the elderly.

Closely related to occupation and income level is the educational level of the population. Since a large component of the public health nurse's practice consists of public health education, an assessment of the educational status of the population helps determine effective educational strategies. Educational level is also an indication of the amount of existing knowledge about disease prevention and the extent to which health concepts will be accepted and understood. Education, similar to income, needs to be evaluated in relation to the context. In some communities, a high school education is meaningful and will be the standard for the community's most prominent citizens, while in others it may represent the very lowest.

Residential and Household Characteristics

BOX #3.18

- **What percentage of the population over age 16 is currently single, married, divorced, widowed?**

- **What is the number of family units in the community?**

- **What is the average population per household?**

- **What is the percentage of single people in the community?**

- **How many households are owner-occupied?**

- **How many households are tenant-occupied?**

- **What percentage of the population lives in substandard housing?**

Different kinds of household configurations distinguish neighborhoods and communities. The prevailing domestic units may consist of young singles or old singles, single parents and their children, grandparents and grandchildren, or any number of combinations in addition to the conventional nuclear family.

Since the household generally is the unit of personal healthcare in the community, it is important for the public health nurse to know how many such units are in the district. This figure is almost, if not equally, as useful to the public health nurse as population size. A nurse serving a population of 3,000, divided into 500 households, will have a practice very different from the nurse serving the same size population, divided into 1,500 households. One-person households, for example, present special challenges, especially if the person is in the senior-citizen age group. Since public health nurses rely on household members to participate in the care of aged or chronically ill residents, many have established innovative alert systems so residents who live alone can watch over one another through daily phone calls or visits.

Households that are too crowded or in substandard condition also place their members at risk for a variety of physiological and psychological health problems and perpetuate health disparities. Since most people spend $\frac{1}{3}$ to $\frac{2}{3}$ of their lives at home, housing will have a profound influence on the health of the population, including the growth and development of children and family functioning. Depending on the type of community, the number of people living in owner-occupied housing as opposed to renter-occupied housing is an indication of the stability and investment of community residents. Those who own real property have a vested interest in keeping up standards of health and safety and in making the community a wholesome place in which to live. Renters often have a lower investment in the community, both economically and emotionally. Therefore, it may be difficult to generate the same intensity of support and enthusiasm for community-based healthcare action from a primarily renting population. Again, however, the extent to which this general rule is expressed in specific communities depends on several factors, and there are many well-known exceptions where renters have rallied on behalf of their community.

MANAGING POPULATION DATA

The analysis of the data collected about the population of a community generally begins with a cross tabulation of its various demographic characteristics. Looking at the relationship between age and sex, and how that relationship will influence health and illness, will help predict future health problems. It is also useful to examine the relationship between age and education, income and residence, age and occupation, sex and occupation, income and family size, and age and residence. In fact, there is an unlimited number of relationships that could be examined, all of which have implications for the health of the community and the delivery of health services. The ones selected should be the ones most useful for solving a particular health problem in a particular community. If, for instance, the goal is to provide flu immunization to all elderly residents, the sites selected should have access to the greatest number of elderly citizens. The critical variable to correlate would, of course, be age, but perhaps an exploration of the role of churches in serving as a site for a program is more important. Therefore, it is important to know the relationships between religious affiliation and age. The community health nurse might also want to know the relationship between residence and age and ethnicity and age. Do most of the elderly live in one section of the community? Do they represent a particular ethnic and/or religious group? The analysis of population data can provide some of the more complex, but also useful, information for understanding the relationships between demographic characteristics and health status.

THE COMMUNITY AS A SOCIAL SYSTEM

The third component of a cultural assessment is a view of the community as a social system. The very term *community* implies people are linked in identifiable ways, including by social institutions that transmit values and culture of the community from one generation to the next. *Defining a community as an aggregate of people who are located in a spatial/temporal environment and linked to one another in a social system* will identify the way in which individual residents and groups in the community relate to one another. In the *Healthy People 2010* document, the social environment is highlighted as one of the six determinants of health. The *social environment* is defined as interactions with family, friends, and others, and as encompassing social institutions. "The social environment has a profound effect on individual health, as well as on the health of the larger community, and is unique because of cultural customs; language; and personal, religious or spiritual beliefs" (USDHHS, 2001, p. 19). There are many ways to describe the social system of a community. The three that have been found to be especially useful in public health, particularly when used together, are (a) community institutions, (b) horizontal stratification of the community, and (c) vertical segmentation of the community (Arensberg, 1954, 1955).

COMMUNITY INSTITUTIONS

Institutions are standardized patterns of social behavior typified by a regular cycle of activities, specific groupings and personnel, and an accompanying set of rules and ideology (Nadel, 1964). The presence and ongoing functioning of institutions give a community its character and its sense of permanence. When an activity or social behavior is "institutionalized," it means it is no longer dependent on a specific person or persons to make it happen, but that it has taken on a life of its own. The institution of marriage is a good example. It is not something each individual invents as he or she reaches adulthood. It is an established social pattern, and though each person has a choice of whether or not to partake in the institution of marriage, it is nonetheless clearly established as a normative expectation of adult life in our society. Marriage has a set of rules, both formal and informal, that govern its performance. Formal rules relate, for example, to who can marry, the age at which a person can become married without parental consent, or who can officiate at a marriage. Less formal rules, on the other hand, might govern the appropriate age difference between the marriage partners or who may be invited to the wedding.

Because something is institutionalized does not mean it is incapable of change. It simply means change will require some kinds of societal reorganization. Using the same example, it is easy to see the institution of marriage has undergone remarkable change with-

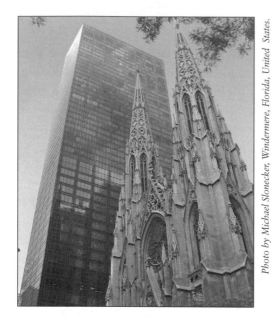

Photo by Michael Slonecker, Windermere, Florida, United States.

in the past 30 years. These changes include, for instance, the age at which many people are choosing to marry, the ease with which a di-vorce is obtained, the roles each of the partners assumes, or the number of times people are married. Moreover, new institutions are always developing to meet societal needs that currently are not being addressed by existing institutions. The changing pattern of marriage in our society has created a need for standardized ways of dealing with divorce and the custody of children. Because divorce was less

common in the past, the activities and behaviors surrounding divorce were not standardized, and each couple was left to work out a solution in their own way, on their own terms.

While contemporary American society values this kind of personal freedom, the absence of societal endorsement of behavior can leave individuals vulnerable to conflict, indecision, personal guilt, and animosity. In recent years, as divorce has become more commonplace, standardized procedures and societal expectations emerged, which help serve to guide both courts and families. Institutionalization offers societal confirmation and serves as an organizing function for a society and its members. For example, societies have institutionalized ways of dealing with death in which expected behavior, routine social support, and a guiding ideology assist families through the bereavement process.

The community assessment boxes presented in this chapter do not cover all institutions that constitute a community's culture, but only the major categories of institutions that one is likely to find in almost all communities. They also are the ones most useful for guiding public health nursing practice and include economic, political and governmental, domestic and family, educational, religious, and recreational and artistic institutions. Depending on the community, different institutions assume different levels of significance, and some institutions not mentioned here may emerge as highly important. The critical factor is not a detailed account of every institution, but the ability to identify institutions and analyze their relationship to the health of the community. Health-related institutions have been omitted, intentionally, from this section because they will be discussed in detail in Chapter 4, which focuses exclusively on health and healthcare.

Economic Institutions

BOX #3.19

- **What is the major economic base of the community (e.g., manufacturing, industrial, wholesale, retail, resort, education, health, government center, commercial center, diversified)?**

- **Describe the relationship between employers and employees or workers and management.**

- **Who are the major employers?**

- **Is there a union? If so, what role does it play?**

- **What changes have taken place in the economy over the past 10 years?**

- **What effect have these economic changes had on the community?**

- **Describe the health and safety factors associated with local industry.**

Like all institutions, the economic institutions of a community can be viewed both as cultural capital and as cultural liability. Economic leaders can be powerful allies in making communities healthy places in which to work, raise families, live in quality housing, receive an education, and grow old comfortably. At the same time, the health of a community may be endangered by an economy grounded in exploitation of specific populations, creating social and health disparities, or grounded in the degradation of the environment and natural resources. The extent to which economic opportunity, such as employment and financing, is available to all sectors of the population is an indication of the economic health of the community. It provides a critical foundation for community health and the elimination of health disparities. Understanding the economy that fuels community life and the changes that have taken place over the years permits the most fundamental understanding of current and future health problems. These phenomena range from potentially dangerous ecological changes and environmental hazards to the physical, psychological, and social problems associated with under- or unemployment (Ratner, 1993; Worthman & Kohrt, 2005). An assessment of health and safety factors of the local economy comprises two components. First is its impact on the environment, including air, noise, water, and food pollution. Second is the direct influence on the health of citizens, including the conditions of employment, income, financial stress, and socioeconomic dislocations.

In some communities, it is relatively easy to describe the local economy and its influence on community health, particularly if it has a single economic base—for example, a farming village, a tourist resort, or a manufacturing town. In others, however, it may take several months or even years to understand a community's economy. Many immigrant populations support their communities of origin with monthly remittances to relatives. Similarly, communities may have an "underground" economy based on activities such as gambling or the sale of illicit drugs. The economic significance of such activities might, in fact, underlie much of the failure to reduce drug abuse in inner cities (Bourgois, 1993). It is now known that illicit drug use and commerce comprise part of a much larger problem, centered around the lack of economic opportunity, that must be addressed before significant strides in the reduction of drug abuse can occur (Dreher, 1982).

Government, Politics, and Law Enforcement

BOX #3.20

- **What is the formal structure of the local government?**

- **What is the government's source of public revenue (e.g., property tax, sales tax)?**

- **What is the process for elections?**

- **Who are the elected representatives for the community?**

- **What political parties are represented and in what proportion?**

- **What is the law enforcement system for the district?**

- **What are the characteristics of the penal system (e.g., jails)?**

- **What local government departments and officials are responsible for overseeing the health of the community?**

- **What proportion of the local government's budget is allocated to health?**

- **What are the voting records of elected officials on health issues?**

It is impossible to guide the health of a community without an understanding of local government. This begins by determining (a) the formal structure of the local government, e.g., town, county, village, municipal, state, district; (b) who has the authority to make decisions on behalf of the community—a president, king, mayor, council, commission, tribal elders, paramount chiefs, etc.; and (c) how the laws and policies created by government are enforced in the community.

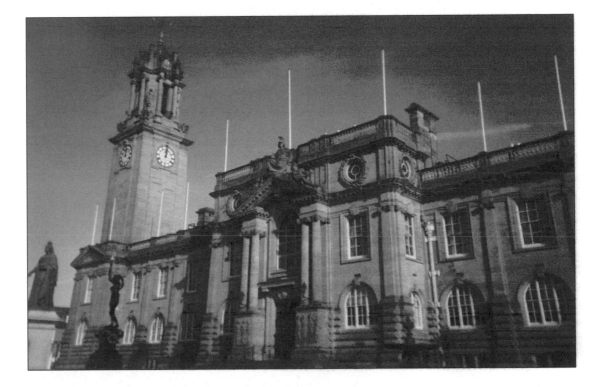

But knowing the system of government is insufficient without knowledge of local politics. Politics, often defined simply as the allocation of scarce resources, influences the direction of government and the way in which government work gets accomplished, as well as who becomes the leaders and the officials. Government is the structure and politics is the process that bends and twists and reshapes official policies in accordance with the local context. Politics is a system of social relations in which access to and exercise of power are played out, where power is defined most elementally as the ability to influence (French & Raven, 1955). While politics exists at every level of human organization, it is at the local level of government that people feel the effects most keenly. This is where governmental decisions and policies enter lives on a daily basis, and where people are most likely to take action—for example, the schools their children attend, the roads on which they drive, the police protection they receive, how their property is zoned, how waste is removed and sanitized, and the taxes they pay are all determined by local government decisions.

The identity of local public officials, how authority was invested in them (elected, appointed, inherited), and their voting records on issues of health and welfare are essential types of information for community health practitioners, both for explaining current health issues and for mobilizing the community for future health action. Political parties may or may not be represented at the most local level, and it is not uncommon to have two or three independent candidates running for office, each with his or her individual agenda and constituency. Of course, there are many communities with a dominant political party affiliation that party leaders acknowledge through governmental assistance in return for community-wide support for the party candidates.

The tax structure, where economic institutions and political institutions come together, is a significant issue for both planning and sustaining a community's health. The concern of citizens over an increasing tax burden created by government initiatives—no matter how wholesome—is very real and can be a major deterrent in planning and implementing a healthy community agenda. The scattering of nuclear power plants throughout the northeast corridor of the United States in previous decades, for example, provided badly needed employment opportunities and tax relief to the citizens of small towns. Thus, while this trend generated some local resistance, centered mainly on health and safety hazards for future generations, the short-term advantages were difficult to counter.

Domestic Organization

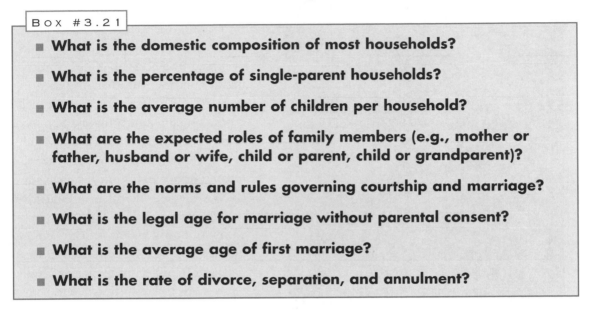

BOX #3.21

- **What is the domestic composition of most households?**

- **What is the percentage of single-parent households?**

- **What is the average number of children per household?**

- **What are the expected roles of family members (e.g., mother or father, husband or wife, child or parent, child or grandparent)?**

- **What are the norms and rules governing courtship and marriage?**

- **What is the legal age for marriage without parental consent?**

- **What is the average age of first marriage?**

- **What is the rate of divorce, separation, and annulment?**

While nursing has endorsed the family as a significant unit of health service, nurses cannot assume all communities are composed of families, or that the constituent families consist of a husband and wife and their unmarried children. Many people tend to use the terms household and family synonymously. Indeed, in our society, they often refer to the same group of people. For the purposes of this community cultural assessment, however, they will be discussed as two separate entities. *Family* will refer to those related by kinship ties, whether by blood, adoption, or marriage; *household* will refer to those who share a living space. While these are grossly oversimplified definitions, it is easy to immediately see that depending on how family is defined, it is possible to have households comprising more than one family and families comprising more than one household. To understand domestic organization, it is better to temporarily set aside a definition of family and instead try to determine what categories of people occupy a household or continuous households. Much of this information is available in census reports.

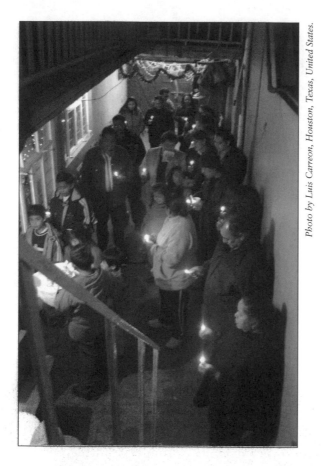

Photo by Luis Carreon, Houston, Texas, United States.

Communities differ greatly in the way their populations are organized into families and households. Some are divided into single household units, occupied by nuclear families consisting of a mother, a father, and their unmarried children. Others are much more complex and contain a variety of domestic arrangements. Extended families may occupy several households located in proximity, with much routine visiting among them. A contrasting pattern prevails in migrant worker communities, where it is not uncommon to have several unrelated individuals and families occupying the same household. It is also possible to have a community in which most individuals live either alone or with an unrelated person, geographically distant from their families. In each case, the problems and strengths are different and must be taken into consideration.

In community health, the household is equally as important as the family. This is ordinarily the unit that eats and sleeps together and has the most routine contact. It is common for household members to have mutual caregiving functions, although it is not at all unusual for these functions to be shared by family members and others who are not part of the household. Since the household generally is the unit of personal healthcare, it is useful to determine what trends are evident in the community's domestic organization. Is there an increase in the divorce rate? Are people marrying later? Are they having fewer children? Is the proportion of single-parent families on the increase? What are the implications of these trends for the kinds of health problems and the delivery of health services?

The roles and ideologies governing family, marital, and domestic life underpin some of our most ingrained institutions. Though it may be difficult, it is imperative for nurses to step away from their own cultural concepts of family and look at domestic organization of the community in an objective and neutral way. For example, rather than deciding in advance that the children of divorced parents are necessarily disadvantaged, it may be more helpful first to determine whether "single-parent families" aren't really "two-household families," in which children divide their time between two households with loving and protective parents. Moreover, in those situations where there is only one parent, surrogate mothers and fathers often emerge from among friends, relatives, and neighbors to create a more healthful psychological environment than that which existed when the biological parents occupied the same household.

Another kind of family structure that has emerged over the past 2 decades is that of same-sex couples who have publicly declared their commitment and live together, sometimes having or adopting children. Most recently, the right of same-sex couples to marry or form civil unions has been a significant issue, both socially and politically. Because the level of social acceptance of a gay sexual orientation has been uneven, *Healthy People 2010* contains a statement that includes sexual orientation as another of the six areas in which health disparities occur. For gay men, health issues include HIV/AIDS, substance abuse, depression, and suicide, while for lesbian women, some evidence points to higher rates of smoking, alcohol abuse, obesity, and stress. For both groups, personal safety and mental health are important issues (USDHHS, 2001).

While the norms of Western society dictate that courting, marriage, and pregnancy proceed in that order, this sequence has changed over the past decades, even if the norms haven't. Norms in other cultures, however, can be quite different; it should not be surprising if marriage is arranged without the benefit of a courtship, or if pregnancy occurs without the benefit of marriage. In fact, in some cultures of the world, it is not uncommon to attend a marriage in which all the children of the couple are part of the wedding party. Traditions that may appear exotic are supported in many ways in the social organization of the community and make sense when understood in their local context (McElroy & Townsend, 2004).

Religious Institutions

BOX #3.22

- **List, by denomination, the churches, temples, and other places of worship attended by residents in the community.**

- **What is the size and average attendance of each congregation?**

- **Which churches are increasing in membership and which are decreasing?**

- **List the names of the clergy for the various churches.**

- **What role does each religious facility play in the healthcare of the community?**

- **What churches have taken leadership positions for neighborhood or community health activity?**

- **Are there religious minority groups in the community?**

Because healthcare has its origins in religious institutions, it remains heavily influenced by religion, both in the organization and delivery of services and as a vehicle of social and psychological support for the participants. While many of the earlier functions in the direct care of the sick have disappeared, some religious groups or functionaries remain strong community advocates for health. Examples include hospital care, psychological counseling, family counseling, senior citizen health promotion programs, and care of children (Magilvy & Brown, 1997; Simington, Olson, & Douglass, 1996). In large cities, where there is a choice of hospitals and other health facilities, many people prefer and actively seek a hospital of their religious affiliation, so they can observe dietary laws and have access to clergy of their own denomination.

In addition to attending to the spiritual needs of their congregations, many religious institutions play a significant role in reducing health disparities through support of their members with money, equipment, medicine, and support services such as cooking, housekeeping, or just visiting sick members and their families. Even if they do not participate directly, religious institutions often lend their facilities to community health services such as after-school programs for teenagers, child day-care centers, senior centers, and sites for health fairs. As do other institutions, organized religions not only have buildings and activities, they also have leaders and officials who are likely to have considerable influence in the community and can support particular health projects. Churches are key institutions for public health because of the active role they take, or can be persuaded to take, in resolving community health problems (Peterson, Atwood, & Yates, 2002). Since 1984, when it began as a form of community-based nursing practice, parish nursing has expanded to 48 states, Canada, Australia, and Korea. As a form of public health nursing practice, parish nursing focuses on health promotion and disease prevention through the roles of health educator, counselor, referral source, advocate, and facilitator. Its distinction lies in the connection between parish nurses and a specific religious denomination and its commitment to interpret the close relationship between faith and health (Brudenell, 2003; McDermott, Solari-Twadell, & Matheus, 1998).

Religion and health often are intertwined and expressed in dietary habits, health-seeking behavior, responses to medical advice, sexual behavior, psychological factors, family relationships, attitudes about death and disability, relationships with health professionals, and even recreational activities. Religious beliefs provide direction for how one responds to health-related behaviors involving diet, pregnancy, family planning, and terminal illness, and must be given consideration in community health education and program development. Furthermore, certain religions may impose injunctions on common screening procedures such as drawing blood, or they may reject scientific explanations of health and disease and require that the nurse reconstruct health programs and interpretation within a more culturally acceptable framework. It is important to know the predominant religions, religious celebrations, and holy days of the population for the appropriate scheduling and timing of health services. Finally, the relationship between religiosity and mortality, suggested 20 years earlier in the Alameda County Study by Berkman and Syme (1979), has been confirmed, with continued lower mortality rates for frequent religious attendees. This appears to be

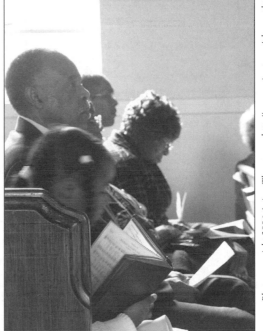

Photo copyright 2006 Anissa Thompson. http://www.anissat.com/photos.php .

explained by improved health practices, increased social contacts, and more stable marriages, which occur in conjunction with attendance (Strawbridge, Cohen, Shema, & Kaplan, 1997).

Educational Institutions

BOX #3.23

- **Under what authority does the school system operate?**

- **Identify pre-college-level schools that serve the population—both public and private.**

- **What is the approximate enrollment in each school or program?**

- **Describe the administration of the local public school system.**

- **What is the function of the school board?**

- **What is the composition of the school board, and how are members elected or appointed?**

- **How is the superintendent of schools selected?**

- **Identify the principal and teachers of each school.**

- **How are school health and nursing services organized?**

- **What other special services are offered in the schools (e.g., psychological counselor, dental hygienist, social worker)?**

- **What educational institutions are used for adult learning in the community (e.g., adult education classes, community colleges, 4-year colleges and universities)?**

- **Identify the libraries and other educational facilities available to community residents.**

The school system is an essential component of a community's cultural capital regarding children's health. In addition to traditional screening in the form of physical, vision, and hearing exams, health promotion is also carried out in schools, with educational programs such as drug abuse prevention, sex education, dental health, nutrition, and hygiene. School records on absenteeism provide an excellent source of data for case finding and epidemiological investigations.

Community practice nurses can begin by locating the schools and educational facilities on a map. School schedules and educational events should be recorded on a community health calendar. By knowing the teachers and their various areas of expertise, and developing relationships with them, community nurses can conveniently and efficiently reach most of the children in a given community. They can help teachers to (a) recognize symptoms of disease, child abuse, and auditory or visual impairment; (b) monitor children with chronic diseases such as diabetes; and (c) provide first aid coverage in the event of emergencies. Most states mandate the employment of a school nurse at both the elementary and secondary levels. The role of the school nurse encompasses the totality of the school health program, incorporating primary, secondary, and tertiary prevention strategies. In addition to providing some personal health services to schoolchildren, school health nurses are charged with creating a healthy school environment that provides a safe, supportive social and learning milieu for all children.

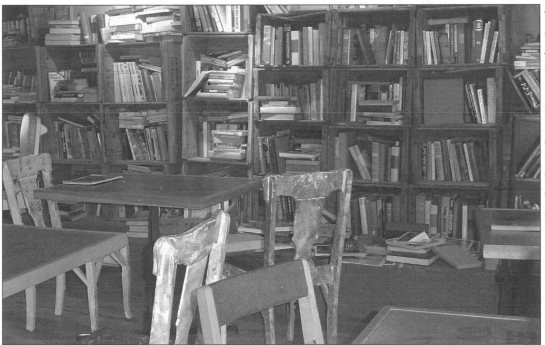

Photo by Alain Fradette, St-Germain, Quebec, Canada.

School boards differ in the degree of influence they exert on schools. Some are very controlling, while others leave the administration to the principal and limit their input to financial matters. The composition and philosophy of the board will influence school health programs, as well as academic programs. In addition to getting to know the principal and teachers, it is important for community health practitioners to become acquainted with board members, identifying those who will be supportive of certain issues and those who will be obstructive.

Adult education classes have become increasingly popular and provide an effective mechanism for offering health-related courses such as emergency care, parenting, and stress reduction. Institutions of higher learning generally are a valuable resource for community nurses. Because they often employ faculty who are experts in various aspects of health and healthcare, they can assume a leadership role in promoting a healthy community agenda.

Because high educational levels strongly correlate with good health status, education is another area highlighted in *Healthy People 2010* as a way to contribute to the prevention of health disparities (USDHHS, 2001). Thus, the effectiveness of our educational systems and the ability of public service workers to reach and teach all members of the community are central to community health.

Recreation

BOX #3.24

- **How do community residents spend their leisure time?**

- **Locate and identify recreational areas and facilities. These include formal recreation facilities (e.g., parks, playgrounds, theaters, zoos, golf courses, public pools) and informal recreational facilities (e.g., streets, vacant lots, swimming holes).**

- **Locate publicly supported facilities, commercial facilities, or age-designated facilities (e.g., children, adolescents, senior citizens).**

- **Where do children play?**

- **What parts of the day and week are generally reserved for leisure activity?**

- **What agencies and personnel are specifically concerned with community recreation and leisure?**

Play and recreation are important components of all societies. Recreation is directly related to health in its capacity for providing exercise, for meeting physical and psychological challenges, and as a form of relaxation and relief of stress. The promotion of organized recreational activities, such as supervised playgrounds and parks, has been a significant healthcare intervention in reducing the incidence of accidents and promoting the safety of children. Recreation generates social interaction in the form of teams and clubs that can break down barriers and create the sense of unity that ultimately limits the disparities in multiethnic or racial communities (Lucas, 1986).

What is typically thought of as recreation must also include books, magazines, radio, videos, and television. As recreational activities, they serve a communication function and are important resources for public health education, particularly in the area of health promotion, prevention of disease, and personal management of health problems. Practically all women's and family magazines have health columns. Television shows, movies, soap operas, and novels deal with a variety of health problems, including driving while intoxicated, teenage suicide, drug abuse, family violence, living with chronic illness, Alzheimer's disease, and death and dying. They are often sensitively written and framed within the cultural experience of the audience. They can be a valuable teaching tool, as well as a vehicle for mobilizing community action. The timing of health education or health screening programs to immediately follow a television drama that has generated the interest of the public can help to ensure its success.

While there are distinct advantages to recreational and leisure facilities for the purpose of promoting the health and safety of community residents, recreational institutions also may generate community health problems. For example, recreational drinking, if not carefully regulated, can have serious consequences for individuals, as well as for the safety of motorists and pedestrians in the community. Monitoring the safety and sanitation of public facilities is another component of community practice. Broken bottles and rusty cans in the park or on a beach can result in serious injuries.

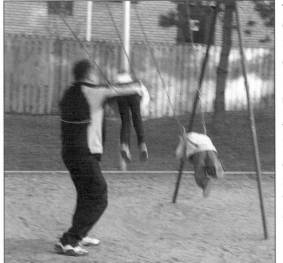

Photo by Matthew Maaskant, Toronto, Ontario, Canada.

Certain leisure activities themselves place the participants at risk of personal injury and therefore require appropriate community resources to both prevent and manage potential injury. While individuals and groups should not be prevented from participating in the pleasures of mountain climbing, scuba diving, running marathons, cycling, football, and so on, risks are often borne by the community as well as the individual if something goes wrong. Winter sports such as snowmobiling, skiing, or skating may require safety declarations, injury prevention programs, and trauma services.

Voluntary Organizations

BOX #3.25

- **Identify the voluntary organizations in the community by type:**
  - **Social**
  - **Economic**
  - **Religious**
  - **Educational**
  - **Political**
  - **Recreational**

- **Identify the leaders of each organization.**

- **Identify informal associations and groups within the community.**

Often public health nurses and other social welfare workers believe part of their work in community development is to establish community councils and committees to help them accomplish their goals for improving the health of the community. While this may be necessary at some point in the community health process, a much more culturally acceptable and efficient way is to take advantage of existing community groups. Voluntary associations represent strength in both leadership and membership that can be readily deployed by community nurses for solving community problems and promoting community health. Each of the institutions already discussed has its own voluntary association consisting of a group of individuals who are bound together by a common interest. However, because these groups are so important to the nurse in mobilizing community action, they are separated here as another form of social institution.

There are many kinds of voluntary associations based on their stated purposes. One category, for example, consists of those based on a common sociodemographic characteristic, such as age (teen groups, young adults), ethnicity (Polish American clubs, Sons of Cuba), attendance at the same school (alumni associations, fraternities and sororities), and so on. Often local branch associations are tied into national organizations and are highly formalized, such as the Masons or Elks clubs. These groups can be an important vehicle for obtaining resources from outside the community.

Typical of economic voluntary associations would be the chamber of commerce, trade associations, professional societies, or Kiwanis clubs. In other cultures, "friendly societies" are economic voluntary associations that assure members a proper funeral and insurance benefits. Occupational groups form to control and oversee various aspects of their trade or profession. Government and political associations, political party branch organizations, and citizens councils usually function to influence legislation locally or nationally or increase access to voting, as in the League of Women Voters. Voluntary associations also may provide protective services such as fire and police protection. Parent-teacher associations are perhaps the best known of all educational voluntary associations, but others include voluntary library service and bookmobiles, as well as travel societies, book clubs, and honor societies.

Organized religion has led the way in establishing lay voluntary associations to carry on community activities. Church brotherhoods or women's committees, YMCA, YWCA, B'nai B'rith, and Jewish community centers are all examples of religious voluntary associations. Many play and artistic activities are also organized on a voluntary basis, including athletic clubs, choruses, bridge clubs, dance and theater groups, and chamber music ensembles.

Voluntary groups ordinarily are formalized with names and charters, regular meetings, and criteria for membership. There may, however, be other groups that are more casual but equally important. These include, for example, the adolescents who routinely meet in the local shopping mall, the elderly who eat breakfast at the same restaurant every morning, and the men who gather each evening on a street corner or play chess in the park. Even though such groups are more difficult to identify, they often have even more influence than formalized groups and provide a constituency that could lend valuable support in creating and implementing a healthy community agenda.

While the stated purpose of each of the voluntary associations may be recreational, religious, educational, economic, or the promotion of ethnic or racial group interests, all voluntary associations serve a number of functions. For example, while social or educational groups are not organized specifically to address political issues, they may have strong lobbying functions and serve as a forum for political expression that would be less meaningful if offered by single individuals. Whether or not their stated objectives are economic, voluntary associations of all kinds have been useful in helping members to acquire jobs, borrow money, and advance in their careers. Holding offices in organizations gives people an opportunity for status and position. Many join voluntary associations as a form of recreation, even if the goals of the association are not recreational. The "friendly societies" mentioned earlier, for example, have a rather somber objective, but regular meetings and outings provide various forms of recreation that further strengthen the social ties among the members.

Voluntary associations are vehicles for newcomers, helping them fit into the community and meet others with similar interests. Often they may substitute for an extended family, providing child care, sick care, and guidance by helping individuals solve personal and domestic problems. Voluntary associations also are vehicles for social control, imposing injunctions on the behavior of members and requiring they conform to specific standards. For example, Alcoholics Anonymous and other self-help groups have blossomed into a panorama of mutual assistance and support, addressing health problems such as obesity, smoking, cancer, muscular dystrophy, diabetes, and Alzheimer's. Many such voluntary associations were inspired and organized on the local level by nurses who recognized that individuals could relate to others with the same problem and learn from them, knowing they had undergone a similar experience.

Horizontal Stratification

BOX #3.26

- **Describe the major socioeconomic levels in the community.**

- **What sociodemographic variables and social institutions distinguish the levels?**

Differences in wealth and status exist in practically all communities, no matter how small and homogeneous they first appear. These differences, when examined at the population level, constitute social classes of people that correlate more or less closely with income, educational level, and occupation. Thus, social class represents categories of people of similar social rank having positions, responsibilities, possessions, and accomplishments of a more or less equal level and value.

For nurses who are unfamiliar with a particular community, patterns of class stratification and socioeconomic differences among residents may be barely distinguishable, particularly if it is a community in which citizens generally have limited access to resources. Indeed, many residents will deny the existence of social classes in their communities, but the recognition of socioeconomic differences is of critical importance in understanding the community social structure and variations in the behavior of residents. The differences that exist on the community level may not always—in fact, often do not—reflect the class differences that exist on the national level. They are nevertheless consequential for the community and are acknowledged by community members. Despite their protestations of equality, they usually have an awareness of their position in relation to others. It is difficult to find a community where differences in status, income, and access to scarce resources do not exist. Even though classes are not formally organized groups, like voluntary associations, they have lives of their own. People enter them through birth or marriage or, with some difficulty, through the acquisition of socioeconomic resources and power as they progress through life. Though there is no formal membership process for entering a class, to be counted one of a specific rank requires that others judge you to be so. This acceptance often is more difficult to obtain than the more formal membership of voluntary associations.

Generally, it is assumed income, family name, occupation, residence, and education guide the social ranking of individuals. However, this is not always the case, and the criteria for determining social rank vary from community to community. Symbols of high social status such as manner of dress, etiquette, residence, and car may be assumed by any member of the community, but they do not mean the person is actually a member of that class. Moreover, such people could be criticized by the upper echelons, as well as their own level, for trying to imitate those of higher social rank. Nor can one automatically assume that a person with money or a profession belongs to a particular social class. Physicians, for example, ordinarily occupy the upper social ranks, but in some of the extremely affluent, "old money" communities of the Northeast US, physicians assume an almost servant class position, respected for their skill and knowledge but not admitted to the upper strata in the social sense.

While the actual ranking of individuals or households in terms of their socioeconomic status is not within the scope of this text, nurses can learn much simply by the way people group themselves for social interaction—particularly in the areas of recreation and education. Indeed, since friendships and social activities often tend to follow class lines, the task of delineating socioeconomic strata for a particular community is not as difficult as one may anticipate. While church memberships may embrace a wide range of social levels, and the workplace may include all ranks present in the community, it is less likely that people of different classes will socialize routinely. The presence of private schools in a community along with the public school system also provides some clues as to how individuals rank themselves and each other. Knowing the social stratification of the community will assist the nurse in identifying and understanding the real power structure of the community that may underlie other structures, such as government. In general, most people in the upper strata of the community also will have greatest access to resources and thus wield considerable power. The support of such people is extremely helpful to the nurse when power and influence are necessary to implement health programs or policies. Such people also can be serious obstacles or threats to community health nurses and must be identified early in the community assessment process.

Vertical Segmentation

BOX #3.27

- **Identify the vertical divisions of the community by type.**

- **Describe them in terms of differences in their institutions and socio-demographic characteristics.**

In contrast to horizontal stratification, vertical segmentations are those factions in the community not necessarily related to socioeconomic status or classes, but which nevertheless divide the community into subgroups. Depending on the community, these could be based on any one of a variety of features including racial, ethnic, residential, religious, political, or occupational. A familiar example of vertical segmentation is the urban neighborhood composed of two or more dominant subgroups—such as Irish and Italian or African American and Puerto Rican—each of which may express a range of class or socioeconomic differentiation. Even though they may live side by side, the two groups may vote for different political candidates, have different social clubs, participate in different recreational activities, attend different churches, and enjoy a different form of family life. Although they may intermingle on a daily basis, when there is dispute between representatives of the two factions, it is likely they will support their respective racial or ethnic groups.

On the other hand, ethnic and racial groups are rarely homogeneous in membership, with social class, age, race, and religious variations prompting differences in values and lifestyles. Moreover, ethnic boundaries are permeated through marriage and sexual activity, and some residents will claim membership in more than one ethnic or racial group.

Determining the dominance of a specific group membership cannot rest solely on the proportion of the population with a particular background. It also requires the presence of both group leaders and institutions. There is no doubt, however, that the presence of a predominant cultural group in a community can be an extraordinary advantage for public health action, once the cultural rules guiding behavior in that group are translated into practice.

Such vertical segmentation is not limited to ethnic and racial groups. Communities may be divided by residence (apartment dwellers versus homeowners), politics (Republicans versus Democrats), religion (Catholics versus Protestants), etc. Historical conflicts in the United States between farmers and ranchers suggest similar factions based on occupation, as a result of competition for the control of land. In some cases, vertical segmentation is not easily discovered and will take several months of living in the community before it becomes evident. Often factions surface only in times of conflict and therefore are not readily visible until such conflict occurs.

Similar to classes, vertical segments are not formally organized groups in the sense of having a regular charter, membership status, formal leadership, explicit rules of behavior, or routine meetings. Rather, they arise when a group of citizens has something in common that makes them different from another such group within the community. Despite the lack of officers, however, there often is a charismatic leader who is heartily endorsed by other members of the group and who is extremely persuasive. These individuals often are as influential, if not more influential, as the officers of a formal organization or even the powerful upper-class citizens. They are a vital part of community dynamics, because they have the ability to sway large numbers of people and control political elections. They are extremely useful to the public health nurse in mobilizing widespread community support for health programs and in shaping their direction.

Vertical segmentations, as an organizing force in community life, also are expressed in different health problems and different preferences for dealing with them. Community health personnel must be sensitive to these differences and address the needs of both segments. In one community, for example, a rural health center had been funded by the federal government to provide primary care for residents who would otherwise have had to drive a distance of 20 to 40 miles for the nearest medical service. In preparation for the establishment of the center, a survey was sent to all residents to determine their needs and how the clinic could best be used. The results of the survey revealed the differences between the two groups. One group, indicating they would continue to get routine medical care in the nearest urban center, placed the highest priority on emergency treatment (e.g., an X-ray machine, 24-hour coverage), particularly in the winter, when skiing accidents were likely to occur. In contrast, the service most commonly requested by the other group, the majority of whom were the wives of farmers and tradesmen, was a weight reduction program. To solicit the patronage of both groups, the clinic staff implemented both emergency care and weight reduction programs.

MANAGING SOCIAL SYSTEM DATA

For many people, the term community implies relationships of equality among its members. The preceding discussion clearly indicates, however, that communities are, in fact, complex entities, made up of diverse institutions and groups with interests and goals that are sometimes shared and sometimes in conflict. In community practice, the nurse needs to know which segments of the community can be counted on to support a particular project and which cannot. It is also important to know which themes and activities unite community residents of various classes and segments and which separate them. It may be difficult, for example, to change public policy unless all the dominant ethnic and racial groups of a multicultural community support the effort, but dissension among the groups may impede a unity of purpose. There are many ways of handling such problems, which will be discussed in later sections of this book. It is first necessary for the nurse to be aware that such divisions exist.

One of the difficulties public health nurses have in working with social systems data is that community organization and structure, unlike the physical environment and population, are conceptual. A series of diagrams depicting the horizontal stratification and vertical segmentation in relation to each other and to community institutions can be very helpful to illustrate the social system and its points of intersection and cleavage. If, for example, the class structure was diagrammed according to religious institutions, it might be found that in some communities, all social levels attend the same church. This would thus be a point of intersection in the community, that is, a place where the nurse could reach a broad range of community residents, as opposed to a specific segment.

SUMMARY

Even though health status has not been addressed directly, how to determine many things about the health of the community simply by looking at its environment, its people, and its social structure has been discussed. Comparable to the psychosocial assessment of individual patients, this information allows the community health nurse to discover current health problems and predict future ones. The community cultural assessment not only is a guide to determining community weaknesses, but also helps to evaluate the strengths—the cultural capital—that can be mobilized to address them. All of this has been discovered without even looking at health status data. In each area of the cultural assessment, however, the implications of each particular bit of information have been considered as they relate to the health and healthcare of the community's population.

REFERENCES

Abraham, L. (1993). *Mama might be better off dead: The failure of health care in urban America*. Chicago: University of Chicago Press.

Agar, M., & MacDonald, J. (1995). Focus groups and ethnography. *Human Organization, 54*(1), 78-86.

American Public Health Association. (1996). *The definition and role of public health nursing: A statement of APHA Public Health Nursing section*. Washington, DC: Author.

Arensberg, C. (1954). The community study method. *American Journal of Sociology, 60*(2), 109-124.

Arensberg, C. (1955). American communities. *American Anthropologist, 57*, 1143-1162.

Azevedo-Garcia, D., Lochner, K.A., Osypuk, T.L., & Subramanian, S.V. (2003). Future directions in residential segregation and health research: A multilevel approach. *American Journal of Public Health, 93(2), 215-220.*

Bent, K. (2003). "The people know what they want": An empowerment process of sustainable, ecological community health. *Advances in Nursing Science, 26*(3), 215-226.

Berkman, L., & Syme, L. (1979). Social networks, host resistance, and mortality: A nine year follow up study of Alameda County residents. *American Journal of Epidemiology, 102*(2), 186-204.

Bhui, K., Stansfeld, S., McKenzie, K., Karlsen, S., Nazroo, J., & Weich, S. (2005). Racial/ethnic discrimination and common mental disorders among workers: Findings from the EMPIRIC study of ethnic minority groups in the United Kingdom. *American Journal of Public Health, 95(3), 496-501.*

Boone, M. (1989). Capital crime: Black infant mortality in the nation's capital. Newbury Park, CA: Sage.

Bourgois, P. (1993). In search of respect: Selling crack in el barrio (2nd ed.). Cambridge, UK: Cambridge University Press.

Brownson, R., Patrick, L., & Davis, J.R. (Eds.). (1993). *Chronic disease epidemiology and control.* Washington, DC: American Public Health Association.

Brudenell, Ingrid (2003). Parish nursing: Nurturing body, mind, spirit and community. *Public Health Nursing, 20(2), 85-94.*

Butterfield, P. (1990). Thinking upstream: Nurturing a conceptual understanding of the societal context of health behavior. *Advances in Nursing Science, 12*(2), 1-8.

Butterfield, P. (2002). Upstream reflections on environmental health. *Advances in Nursing Science, 21*(1), 32-49.

Carlson, E., & Chamberlain, R. (2004). The black-white perception gap and health disparities research. *Public Health Nursing, 21*(4), 372-379.

Chambers, R. (1985). Shortcut methods of gathering social information for rural development projects. In M. Cernea (Ed.), *Putting people first.* Oxford, UK: Oxford University Press.

Clark, M.J., Cary, S., Dumert, G., Ceballos, R., Sefuentes, M., Atteberry, I., et al. (2003). Involving communities in community assessment. *Public Health Nursing, 20*(6), 456-463.

Craig, C. (1994). Community determinants of health for rural elderly. *Public Health Nursing, 11*(4), 242-246.

Dreher, M. (1982). *Working men and ganja.* Philadelphia: ISHI Publications.

Dressler, W. (1991). *Depression in a Southern black community.* Albany, NY: State University of New York Press.

Dressler, W., Grell, G.A.C., & Viteri, F.E. (1995). Intracultural diversity and the sociocultural correlates of blood pressure: A Jamaican example. *Medical Anthropology Quarterly, 9*(3), 291-313.

Eberhardt, M., & Pamuk, E. (2004). The importance of place of residence: Examining health in rural and non-rural areas. *American Journal of Public Health, 94*(10), 1682-1686.

Ervin, A. (1997). Trying the impossible: Relatively "rapid" methods in a city-wide needs assessment. *Human Organization, 56*(4), 379-387.

French, J.R., & Raven, B.H. (1955). The basis of social power. In D. Cartwright (Ed.), *Studies in social power*. Ann Arbor, MI: University of Michigan Press.

Guralnik, J., & Leveille, S. (1997). Annotation: Race, ethnicity and health outcomes—unraveling the mediating role of socioeconomic status. *American Journal of Public Health, 87*(5), 728-729.

Grim, C., & Wilson, T. (1993). Salt, slavery, and survival: Physiological principles of the evolutionary hypothesis on hypertension among Western Hemisphere blacks. In J. Fray & J. Douglas (Eds.), *Pathophysiology of hypertension in blacks*. Oxford, UK: Oxford University Press.

Harrison, F. (1998). Introduction: Expanding the discourse on "Race." *American Anthropologist, 100*(3), 609-631.

Higgs, Z.R., Boyne, T., & Murphy, D. (2001). Health care access: A consumer perspective. *Public Health Nursing, 18*(1), 3-12.

Hill, C. (1986). *Community health systems in the rural American South*. Boulder, CO: Westview Press.

Holloway, R. (2003). Personal communication. Columbia University Department of Anthropology.

Krieger, N., Chen, J.T., Waterman, P. Rekpopf, D., & Subramanian, S.V. (2005). Painting a truer picture of US socio-economic and racial/ethnic health inequalities: The Public Health Disparities Geocoding project. *American Journal of Public Health, 95*(2), 312-323.

Landrigan, P. (1992). Commentary environmental disease—A preventable epidemic. *American Journal of Public Health, 84*(10), 1691-1692.

Lucas, J.A. (1986). *Common ground. A turbulent decade in the lives of three American families*. New York: Vintage Books

Magilvy, J.K., & Brown, N.J. (1997). Parish nursing: Advanced practice nursing model for healthier communities. *Advanced Practice Nursing Quarterly, 2*(4), 67-72.

Mason, D. (2000). Nursing in the new millennium: Vision, activism, and the role of the media. *Imprint, 47*(3), 44-53.

McDermott, M.A., Solari-Twadell, P., & Matheus, R. (1998). Promoting quality education for the parish nurse and the parish nurse coordinator. *Nursing and Health Care Perspectives, 19*(1), 4-5.

McElroy, A., & Townsend, P. (2004). *Medical anthropology in ecological perspective*. New York: Westview Press

Meleis, A.I., Lipson, J.G., & Paul, S.M. (1992). Ethnicity and health among five Middle Eastern immigrant groups. *Nursing Research, 41*(2), 98-103.

Melnyk, K. (1988). Barriers: A critical review of recent literature. *Nursing Research, 37*(4), 196-201.

Montague, A. (1997). *Man's most dangerous myth: The fallacy of race*. Walnut Creek, CA: Altamira Press.

Mullings, L. (1978). Ethnicity and stratification in the urban United States. *Annals of the New York Academy of Science, 318*, 10-22.

Munhall, P. (1992). Holding the Mississippi River in place and other implications for qualitative research. *Nursing Outlook*, Nov-Dec, 257-262.

Munhall, P. (2002). *Nursing Research: A qualitative perspective*. Sudbury, MA: Jones T. Bartlett Publishers.

Nadel, S.F. (1964). *The foundations of social anthropology*. New York: Free Press of Glencoe.

Needle, R, Trotter, R.T., Singer, M., Bates, C., Page, J.B., Metzger, D., et al. (2003). Rapid assessment of the HIV/AIDS crisis in racial and ethnic minority communities: An approach for timely community interventions. *American Journal of Public Health, 93*(6), 970-979.

Norman, P., Boyle, P., & Rees, P. (2004). Selective migration, health and deprivation: A longitudinal analysis. *Social Science and Medicine, 60*, 2755-2771.

Peterson, J., Atwood, J., & Yates, B. (2002). Key elements for church-based health promotion programs: Outcome-based literature review. *Public Health Nursing, 19*(6), 410-411.

Plescia, M., Koontz, S., & Laurent, S. (2001). Community assessment in a vertically integrated health care system. *American Journal of Public Health, 91*(5), 811-814.

Quad Council of Public Health Nursing Organizations. (2004). Public Health Nursing Competencies. *Public Health Nursing 21*(5), 443-452.

Ratner, M.S. (Ed.). (1993). *Crack pipe as pimp*. New York: Lexington Books.

Rodwin, V., & Neuberg, L. (2005). Infant mortality and income in 4 world cities: New York, London, Paris and Tokyo. *American Journal of Public Health, 95*(1), 86-90.

Sanday, P.R. (1979). The ethnographic paradigms(s). *Administrative Science Quarterly, 24,* 527-538.

Schultz, P.R., & Magilvy, J.K. (1988). Assessing community health needs of elderly populations: Comparison of three strategies. *Journal of Advanced Nursing, 13,* 193-202.

Schulte, J. (2000). Finding ways to create connections among communities: Partial results of an ethnography of urban public health nurses. *Public Health Nursing, 17*(1), 3-10.

Scrimshaw, S., & Hurtado, E. (1987). *Rapid assessment procedures for nutrition and primary health care.* Los Angeles: UCLA Latin American Center Publications.

Simington, J., Olson, J., & Douglass, L. (1996). Promoting well-being within a parish. *Canadian Nurse, 92*(1), 20-24.

Singh, G.K., & Yu, S.M. (1995). Infant mortality in the United States: Trends, differentials, and projections, 1950 through 2010. *American Journal of Public Health, 85*(7), 957-965.

Sorlie, P., Backlund, E., & Keller, J.B. (1995). U.S. mortality by economic, demographic, and social characteristics: The National Longitudinal Mortality Study. *American Journal of Public Health, 85*(7), 949-956.

Stevens, P. (1996). Focus groups: Collecting aggregate-level data to understand community health phenomena. *Public Health Nursing, 13*(3), 170-176.

Strawbridge, W., Cohen, R., Shema, S., & Kaplan, G. (1997). Frequent attendance at religious services and mortality over 28 years. *American Journal of Public Health, 87*(6), 957-961.

Swinney, J., Anson-Wonkka, C., Maki, E., & Corneau, J. (2001). Community assessment: A church, community and the parish nurse. *Public Health Nursing, 18*(1), 40-44.

Templeton, A. (1998). Human races: A genetic and evolutionary perspective. *American Anthropologist, 100*(3), 632-650.

Urrutia-Rojas, X., & Aday, L.A. (1991). A framework for community assessment: Designing and conducting a survey in a Hispanic immigrant and refugee community. *Public Health Nursing, 6*(4), 163-168.

U.S. Department of Health and Human Services. (2001). *Healthy people 2010.* McLean, VA: International Medical Publishing.

Wolf, E. (1994). Perilous ideas: Race, culture, people. *Current Anthropology, 35*(1), 1-12.

Worthman, C.M., & Kohrt, B. (2005). Receding horizons of health: Biocultural approaches to public health paradoxes. *Social Science and Medicine, 61*, 861-878.

4

COMMUNITY HEALTH ASSESSMENT

The measure of a healthy community is not the complete absence of problems but how well the community prepares for and responds to them.

In the previous chapter, the identification and examination of health were temporarily set aside to concentrate on knowing the community in all its various parameters—its strengths and challenges, and the availability of cultural capital for building community capacity. Although it was possible to identify actual and potential health problems simply by examining the environment, population, and social organization, the appraisal of health and the health system was largely circumspect. Now it is time to conduct a focused assessment of the *health* status of the community's population and environment and the infrastructure dedicated to the pursuit of health.

CHAPTER 4 OBJECTIVES

- Identify sources of population health assessment data.
- Interpret health data using biostatistician and epidemiological measures.
- Determine the health status of the population.
- Examine the health of the environment.
- Identify the cultural capital dedicated to the pursuit of health.
- Compare the community's health institutions in terms of primary, secondary, and tertiary prevention.

WHAT IS A HEALTHY COMMUNITY?

Even the most ideal communities are subject to factors that are either uncontrollable or unforeseeable—a flu epidemic, the aging of a population, or natural disasters such as hurricanes, tornadoes, or earthquakes. The measure of a healthy community, then, is not the complete absence of problems, but rather how well the community prepares for and responds to them. Thus, the parameters of what constitutes a healthy community must include the cultural capital required to anticipate and manage the problems that inevitably will emerge. The goal of a community health assessment is to identify not only the challenges, but also the strengths embedded in the community's environment, social structure, and population. This information enables community nurses to mobilize individuals and social institutions to design and implement interventions that will ameliorate health problems and decrease risk.

The health assessment schedule that follows is not exhaustive. Like the assessment boxes provided in Chapter 3 to inventory the community's *culture*, it includes a common set of inquiries used to describe and analyze a community's *health*. Depending on the community, some data will be more useful than others, and additional data may be needed to understand and address specific health problems.

While measures of disease, death, and health status are useful vital signs and symptoms of a population's health, a community's health is not simply the aggregate of the health status of its individual citizens (Chapter 2). Rather, the true measure of health is its capacity t extend the quality and years of healthy life for its citizens and eliminate health disparities (U.S. Department of Health and Human Services [USDHHS], 2001). A healthy community is one that is grounded in a wholesome environment, promotes social justice and inclusiveness, and prevents and responds to health risks and problems in a timely and culturally sensitive manner.

MEASURING THE HEALTH OF COMMUNITIES

Traditionally, the health of communities was measured almost exclusively by the presence or absence of disease in its population, especially acute, infectious disease. Epidemiology, originally the study of epidemics, has been expanded to include chronic illness and other health problems such as crime rates, automobile injuries, substandard housing, high school graduation rates, and health disparities. A goal of epidemiological research is to identify the risk factors associated with prevailing public health problems. Based on this research, screening programs are implemented for early detection of these risk factors (e.g., high cholesterol levels, low birth weight, child abuse) and early intervention. Epidemiological research also identifies populations, known as high-risk groups, particularly vulnerable to specific illnesses. Risk groups can be associated with many kinds of factors, such as biological (breast cancer in women), ethnic (diabetes in some Native American groups), socio-economic (high rates of asthma in children of families below the poverty level), occupational (chemical exposure in the workplace), and lifestyle (cigarette smoking). *Healthy People 2010* has established leading health indicators to highlight these vulnerablities (See Table 1).

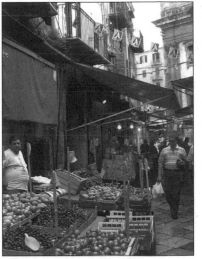

Photo by Alex Zhavoronkova, Rome, Italy.

In addition to morbidity and mortality statistics—commonly used to assess the level of death, disease, and disability in populations—*Healthy People 2010* has identified other areas (**Table 3**) that attempt to measure health. Some of these areas, such as quality of life, are more subjective and difficult to measure than disease and death, but are some of the only evaluations that truly reflect well-being. *Healthy People 2010* endorses three such indicators: a global sense of well-being, days of poor physical or mental health, and the difference between life expectancy and years of healthy life (USDHHS, 2001).

TABLE 1   LEADING HEALTH INDICATORS

Physical Activity
Overweight and Obesity
Tobacco Use
Substance Abuse
Responsible Sexual Behavior
Mental Health
Injury and Violence
Environmental Quality
Immunization
Access to Healthcare

(U.S. Department of Health and Human Services, 2001)

The identification and elimination of population risk factors and the implementation of primary and secondary prevention for high-risk groups have been priorities in community health nursing. Not all health problems, however, fit neatly into this paradigm of high-risk factors and groups. No one is exempt from the common cold, for example.

Moreover, the identification of high-risk groups has been highly criticized for fostering prejudice and discrimination aimed at specific groups, such as gay men at risk for AIDS, rather than attending to the problem behavior, i.e., unprotected sex (Farmer, 1992; Glick-Schiller, 1992). This focus on group identity rather than behavior as the risk factor often has resulted in "blaming the victim" and is a serious deterrent to understanding and addressing health disparities (Galanter, 1977). Even focusing on the health of populations with the goal of changing behavior, for example, exercise programs, smoking cessation, or screening protocols, often has distracted community health nurses from the large-scale environmental and social actions that would address the sources of these unhealthy behaviors.

Examining the community infrastructure as a source of health is consistent with the mandates of *Healthy People 2010,* which underscores environmental and structural factors as critical for monitoring and evaluating health status (USDHHS, 2001; Tables 2 & 3). A variety of structural indicators has been identified that reveal the health disparities associated with social class, income, education, ethnicity, or race (Blane, 1995; Howard, Anderson, Russell, Howard, & Burk, 2000; Singh & Yu, 1995; Steenland, Hu, & Walker, 2004; Woolf, Johnson, Fryer, Rust, & Satcher, 2004). Most of these indicators have typically not been included in health status measures, but they are linked to the 467 Healthy People 2010 objectives that target specific areas for improvement and require routine monitoring. Thus while many measures relate to socio-demographic factors, e.g., the socioeconomic status and educational levels of the population, others reflect community infrastructure and the use and distribution of health and social resources. There are, in fact, infinite ways to measure the health of a community; the most comprehensive assessment properly makes use of a broad range of indicators that include measures of the population, measures of the environment, and measures of the way they interact.

TABLE 2 *HEALTHY PEOPLE 2010* FOCUS AREAS

Access to Quality Healthcare
Arthritis, Osteoporosis, Chronic Back Conditions
Cancer
Chronic Kidney Disease
Diabetes
Disability and Secondary Conditions
Educational and Community-Based Programs
Environmental Health
Family Planning

Food Safety
Health Communication
Heart Disease and Stroke
HIV
Immunization and Infectious Diseases
Injury and Violence Prevention
Maternal, Infant, and Child Health
Medical Product Safety
Mental Health and Mental Disorders
Nutrition and Overweight
Occupational Safety and Health
Oral Health
Physical Activity and Fitness
Public Health Infrastructure
Respiratory Diseases
Sexually Transmitted Infections
Substance Abuse
Tobacco Use
Vision and Hearing

(U.S. Department of Health and Human Services, 2001)

TABLE 3 *HEALTHY PEOPLE 2010* AREAS FOR MONITORING AND EVALUATING HEALTH STATUS

Birth Rates
Death Rates
Life Expectancy
Quality of Life
Morbidity Rates
Risk Factors
Utilization of Health Services
Accessibility of Health Services
Financing of Healthcare
And Many More

(U.S. Department of Health and Human Services, 2001)

ANALYZING THE HEALTH OF COMMUNITIES

Like the community cultural assessment, the community health assessment has an analytical component as well as a descriptive component. The occurrence and distribution of environmental and social problems, as well as the occurrence of death and disease, are analyzed by (1) comparing them with similar groups across time and populations, and (2) tracing them against the backdrop of place and time, population characteristics, and social structure. The second, more qualitative analysis also helps identify patterns and determine risk factors; for example, the preponderance of chronic lung disease in a particular neighborhood, the increase in traffic accidents on Friday evenings, or female employees being more affected by diseases of stress than male employees. Thus, the analysis of community health data is based on four questions similar to those presented in Chapter 3 in the analysis of community cultural data.

■ How do the data vary with time? For example, how does the current incidence of domestic violence compare with the previous 5 and 10 years?

■ How do the data compare with the data of other communities of similar size and type and with local, state, and national findings? For example, how does the community's rate of AIDS compare with the rate of AIDS at the county, state, and national levels?

■ How are the findings regarding the health of the community related to the categories of the community cultural assessment? For example, how are disparities in pregnancy outcome linked to time, place, population characteristics, and social organization?

■ What are the implications of a health problem in one community population on the health of other populations? For example, what effect would alcohol use by adolescents have on other populations in the community?

ASSESSING THE HEALTH OF POPULATIONS

Most people consider themselves members of various groups. These might include ethnic or racial identifications, age categories, geopolitical constituencies, social classes, religion adherents, etc. In fact, all of these classifications have been used at one time or another to categorize people for purposes of public health intervention, research, and analysis. Earlier, reference was made to various biostatistical measures that describe events at the population level—birth rates, death rates, or rates of lung cancer—and to epidemiological studies used to determine the causes of disease, death, and disability.

Using rates, rather than raw numbers, enables the comparison of one group with another to discover differences in health status between and among populations. After differences are found, the next step is to ask why. Why is the rate of infant mortality different from one community to another? Among racial and ethnic groups? Between teenagers and adults? Although less easy to discover, it is not very different from asking why a patient has a temperature higher or lower than the average body temperature.

The discussion in this section will include the commonly established categories to which rates refer, the standard divisions into which public health rates often are framed, and where they can be accessed. In addition, this section includes an overview of the most common epidemiological strategies used to identify risk factors and at-risk groups.

BIOSTATISTICAL MEASURES OF POPULATION HEALTH

Birth, death (mortality), and illness (morbidity) statistics ordinarily are expressed as rates rather than absolute numbers, because rates enable comparison of the experience of populations with one another, as well as in different time frames. Each rate is computed by dividing the number of events in question, e.g., death by suicide, occurring during a specific time period by the population at risk for the event during the same time period. The phrase "population at risk" means all those members of a population who have the potential for experiencing the health problem in question. For example, since women are not eligible to acquire testicular cancer, they would not be counted among the population at risk for morbidity or mortality for that disease. But since all members of a population have the potential for dying, death rates are usually calculated using the entire population as the denominator.

CALCULATING RATES

The numerator and denominator used in calculating rates must reflect the same population in the same time period, with the numerator being included in the denominator. The number in the denominator is computed by using the population at the midpoint of the specified time period.

$$\text{RATE} = \frac{\text{The number of specified events during a particular time period}}{\text{The population at risk for the event at midpoint during the time period}} \times 1{,}000,\ 10{,}000,\ 100{,}000$$

Rates are expressed as multiples of 100, 1,000, 10,000, or 100,000. The choice of multiplicative factor depends on the size of the population and the frequency with which the event occurs. The rates should be expressed in a figure that is not so small that it must be expressed in a fraction or so large that it is awkward or unwieldy. The mortality rate of AIDS in the early years of the epidemic in the United States was given as a multiple of 1,000,000, for example, as cases were few at that time. Currently the rate is expressed per 100,000, as this reflects the increase in diagnosed cases over the past 20 years.

To express the rate of AIDS for a specific city of 500,000 inhabitants, where there were five reported cases of AIDS, the morbidity rate would be .01 per 1,000, or .1 per 10,000. While both calculations tell us the same thing and thus theoretically could be used interchangeably, 1 per 100,000 is the least cumbersome and most broadly applied. Convention also tends to dictate the multiplicative factor. Infant mortality rates, for example, are commonly expressed using 1,000 as the multiplicative factor, while maternal mortality rates, reflecting a less frequent event, are usually expressed using 10,000. In any case, the multiplicative factor should always be mentioned in reporting the rate.

By looking at the rate, rather than the absolute number of occurrences, groups of different sizes may be compared to determine the relative severity of the problem in any population. For most purposes, raw numbers are not useful in a community health assessment because they do not lend themselves to comparison with other communities and populations, and thus their significance is obscured. In other words, it is impossible to know if the number of cases is low or high relative to other communities or if it represents a major departure from previous numbers for that community.

Crude rates, which have not been adjusted to take age or other factors into account, may yield unwarranted conclusions. For example, it would be misguided to compare the crude death rate in a retirement community with that of a community where elders represent only five percent of the population.

$$\text{CRUDE DEATH RATE} = \frac{\text{The number of deaths}}{\text{Total population}} \times 100,000$$

To make such a comparison, it would be necessary to adjust for the age factor to produce a *standardized rate*, called an *age-adjusted rate*. An age-adjusted rate is calculated by assuming the age distribution in all communities is the same, thus eliminating the confounding factor of age. As age is the single best predictor of overall mortality and morbidity, the age-adjustment of mortality and morbidity rates is crucial for evaluative purposes (Morton, Hebel, & McCarter, 2001). There are many different kinds of rates that can be used to describe the health status of a population; for example, age-specific rates (the rate of teenage death), sex-specific rates (the rate of alcoholism among females), or any other possible subgrouping of a larger population. The denominator in these instances is that number of the total population only in the specified subgroup.

An understanding of statistical rates and how they are calculated is the first step in assessing the health of a community's population. In clinical nursing, a client's "vital signs" provide a gross, but immediate and important indication of his or her well-being. In population assessment, the vital signs are health status indicators that include not only mortality and morbidity rates, but also many of the statistics presented in Chapter 3. For example, poverty rates, unemployment rates, and the percentage of the population on public assistance all help to predict the kinds and amount of health problems in any given population. The Centers for Disease Control and Prevention (CDC) has recommended a standard set of health status indicators to be used by each state. It is critical for public health providers to know whether the state has developed this kind of instrument and how to access it.

Selecting the health status indicators that will provide the most relevant information about the health of a community depends largely on the community and the concerns of its residents. For example, using maternal-child health statistics to measure the well-being of a retirement community would not be very useful. Nor would it be helpful to rely as heavily on chronic disease rates to evaluate the health status of a developing country that is more impacted by infectious diseases.

Mortality Rates

BOX #4.1

- **What are the age-adjusted rates for the five leading causes of death in the community?**

- **How do they compare with the rates for the previous 5 and 10 years?**

- **How do they compare with state and national rates?**

- **What trends and differences are present, and how can they be explained?**

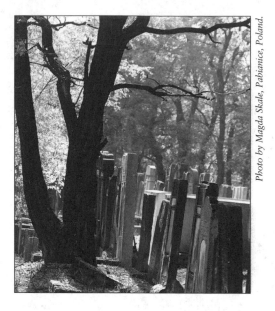

Photo by Magda Skale, Pabianice, Poland.

Mortality rates measure the number and categories of deaths. Crude death rates are based on the entire population, while specific mortality rates relate to the number of deaths in various categories, such as a particular subgroup of the population (e.g., children, an ethnic group) or deaths from specified causes (accidents, cancer). It is not unusual for the top three causes of death in a particular community to be consistent with national statistics. In most states, death rates are highest for cardiovascular disease, cancer, and stroke. It is the remaining seven where most local variation is likely to occur and that provide the most significant information regarding the health status of a particular community.

$$\text{CAUSE SPECIFIC DEATH RATE} = \frac{\text{Total number of deaths from a specified cause}}{\text{Total population}} \times 1{,}000,\ 10{,}000,\ 100{,}000$$

(Crude death rate for a specific cause)

Morbidity Rates

BOX #4.2

- **What are the incidence and prevalence rates of the five leading causes of death in the community?**

- **How do they compare with the rates for the previous 5 and 10 years?**

- **How do they compare with state and national rates?**

- **What trends and differences are present, and how can they be explained?**

- **Which populations are disproportionately affected by infectious disease?**

Unlike mortality rates, which are concerned with the numbers and kinds of deaths in a population, morbidity rates are concerned with the occurrence of various diseases or health problems in a population. Thus the number of people who die from neoplastic disease is reflected in the death rate, while the number of people who are diagnosed with neoplastic disease is expressed in a morbidity rate. Morbidity rates are reported in terms of incidence and prevalence. *Incidence* refers to the number of *newly reported* cases that occur during a specified period of time. *Prevalence*, on the other hand, is more a snap-shot approach and refers to the total number of cases (new and old) that exist in a specified period of time. If, for example, a total of 20 new cases of diabetes had been reported during 2004 in a population of 10,000, the incidence rate for that year would be 2 per 1,000. As those 20 join the ranks of the 180 individuals already diagnosed with diabetes, swelling the total number to 200, the prevalence rate for diabetes in the district would be 20 per 1,000. Occasionally, one sees reference to an *attack rate*. This is a subcategory of the incidence rate and refers to a very limited period of time. For example, one might use the attack rate to measure the effects of an outbreak of salmonella poisoning or measles.

Incidence and prevalence rates have different uses. The purposes of the incidence rate are (a) to determine etiology or causation, and (b) to identify trends in disease occurrence. When the incidence rate rises, this gives cause to suspect that a new etiological agent is operative, *or* that the etiological factors already known have increased in amount or virulence. The prevalence rate, on the other hand, is used to plan for public health services. It gives a current picture of the total number of people who are alive with the illness at a given point in time.

$$\text{INCIDENCE} = \frac{\text{Number of new cases of a disease or health problem occurring during a specified period of time}}{\text{Population at risk at midpoint in time period}} \times 1{,}000,\ 10{,}000,\ 100{,}000$$

$$\text{PREVALENCE} = \frac{\text{Total number of cases of a disease or health problem occurring during a specified time period}}{\text{Total population at midpoint in time period}} \times 1{,}000,\ 10{,}000,\ 100{,}000$$

Increases in the prevalence rate can reflect an increase in incidence plus duration, i.e., there are more cases than usual, or more successful treatment outcomes that result in more people with the illness surviving for longer periods of time. Thus, decreases in the prevalence rate may be due to death or to the discovery of curative treatments. New treatment methods alone do not influence the prevalence rate unless they are successful in curing the illness.

From the size and composition of the population, it is possible to anticipate both the amount and content of health services needed now and in the future. Morbidity data address health problems even more directly and refine predictions of population health status. Both incidence and prevalence rates are important and useful, because they give very different kinds of information about the presence of illness in the community. Unfortunately, they often are difficult to obtain at the local level because they require the population to be surveyed, which is very time-consuming and expensive. Usually, only incidence rates for reportable infectious diseases, such as AIDS, tuberculosis, sexually transmitted infections, and cancer, are available for local communities. In addition, when the total population of a community is very small, the health department often will not publish these rates for privacy reasons.

EPIDEMIOLOGICAL STUDIES OF POPULATION HEALTH

Monitoring the incidence rate is critical for identifying etiology and new causal agents. Since the resources for doing this often are not sufficient, there are epidemiological research strategies that correlate suspected risk factors with the occurrence of disease when the population incidence rates are not available. These research approaches are known as cohort or prospective studies and case-control or retrospective studies.

CASE CONTROL STUDIES

When an agent or factor is suspected of being causally related to the occurrence of a disease, a case-control study (**Table 4**), also referred to as a retrospective study, may be conducted. Case-control studies can be carried out in a reasonably short period of time and are the least expensive. In it, two groups of people—one with the disease and one without—are identified. These groups are further subdivided into those who have been exposed to the suspected etiological agent and those who have not. This comparison yields a statistic called an *odds ratio (OR)*, which calculates the odds of having the disease when the suspected factor is present as opposed to absent.

Some of the most commonly accepted risk factors have been implicated as the result of case-control studies: smoking and lung cancer, family history and breast cancer, high absorbency tampons and toxic shock syndrome. Odds ratios are estimations of a statistic called the *relative risk (RR)*, which can only be calculated when the true incidence rate of a disease is available. The higher the odds ratio or relative risk, the more likely the suspected etiologic factor is causally related to disease incidence. In the case of breast cancer, for example, three factors consistently identified by case-control studies with an odds ratio of greater than four are older age, birth in a North American or northern European country, and having a mother and sister with a history of breast cancer (Cuzick, 2003; Kelsey, 1993). The latter two factors strongly suggest either a genetic or environmental etiology, and in fact, a breast cancer gene has been isolated. Impetus for exploring this genetic line of research was no doubt prompted by the strong association found in many case-control studies that linked breast cancer to family history and country of origin. Other well-publicized risk factors for breast cancer, such as multiparity, early age at menarche, late age at menopause, and alcohol consumption, have lower relative risks—between 1.1 and 2 (Cuzick, 2003; Kelsey, 1993). As none of the risk factors identified to date accounts either alone or together for the majority of breast cancer incidence, other risk factors will need to be studied for their role in breast cancer etiology.

TABLE 4 CASE-CONTROL STUDY

220 women with breast cancer are recruited for a study and are compared with 1,140 women who do not have the disease. The total group is further divided into those with a sister or mother who has breast cancer (exposure present) and those who do not (exposure absent). Typically, a case-control study is depicted in a 2 x 2 table.

		Disease		
		Present	Absent	Totals
Exposure	Present	100(a)	150(b)	250
	Absent	120(c)	990(d)	1100

The equation for establishing an odds ratio is:

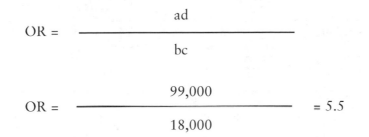

$$OR = \frac{ad}{bc}$$

$$OR = \frac{99,000}{18,000} = 5.5$$

Thus the odds of someone with a mother or sister with breast cancer being diagnosed with the same disease in this sample is 5.5 times greater than for someone without a similar family history.

COHORT STUDIES

When sufficient evidence exists to suggest a link between a factor and a disease, a *cohort* study might be proposed (**Table 5**). This type of study, also referred to as *longitudinal*, examines the disease experience of a cohort of people over time. Cohort studies might be historical, in which the records of large groups of people exposed to a certain risk (for example, workers in an asbestos manufacturing plant) are examined for past level of exposure and disease occurrence. They also can be *prospective*, in which a total population or representative sample is followed over time, and morbidity and mortality rates are related to study variables.

Much of what is known about risk factors for coronary heart disease comes from an ongoing prospective study begun in Framingham, MA, in 1949 (Valanis, 1999). Cohort studies of this type are very useful but often prohibitively expensive. Using the cohort design, a relative risk can be calculated by dividing the incidence rate of a disease among those exposed by the incidence rate among those not exposed. Thus relative risk measures the strength of the association between a factor and an outcome (Morton, Hebel, & McCarter, 2001). Again, the higher the odds ratio or relative risk, the more likely the factor being studied is causal or etiological.

TABLE 5 COHORT STUDY

A group of nurses is followed for 40 years, from first licensure until the present, and the occurrence of lung cancer is recorded. 40,000 nurses are enrolled in the study, and they are divided into smokers and nonsmokers:

Disease

Risk Factor		Lung cancer	No lung cancer	Total
	Smokers	1,400 (a)	14,600 (b)	16,000
	Nonsmokers	200 (c)	23,800 (d)	24,000

The equation for calculating the relative risk is:

$$\text{Relative Risk} = \frac{\text{incidence rate among exposed}}{\text{incidence rate among nonexposed}}$$

Thus in this case the equation reads:

$$RR = \frac{a/(a+b)}{c/(c+d)} = \frac{1,400/16,000}{200/24,000}$$

or

10.5

In this sample, it can be concluded that the probability of developing lung cancer is 10.5 times higher for nurses who smoke than for those who do not smoke.

Causal relationships are demonstrated even more strongly by calculating the difference in disease occurrence in groups exposed to the factor to different degrees—for example, comparing the odds ratios or relative risks from case-control or cohort studies for lung cancer in those who smoked one, two, and three packs of cigarettes a day. If greater exposure results in a higher odds ratio or relative risk, what is called a *dose response relationship* has been established, with causality more likely. In fact, this is exactly how the now widely accepted causal relationship between smoking and lung cancer was established.

The rate and kind of illnesses and disabilities that prevail in a community offer a more refined measure of the health of a population than do birth and death rates. Patterns of morbidity are determined and anticipated not only from incidence rates of reportable infectious diseases, but also from prevalence rates of chronic diseases and disability; maternal-child health indices, such as percentages of pregnant women receiving adequate prenatal care; and rates of mental health and behavioral problems, such as depression, substance abuse, and tobacco smoking.

In the best of all possible worlds, all these data would be readily available and recorded in a format that would encourage comparability over time; between subpopulation groups; and among state, national, and international levels. This is not always the case, however, and it is very important to know where and how to access data for a comprehensive community health assessment.

COMMUNITY HEALTH STATUS: VULNERABLE GROUPS

Life expectancy and health-related quality of life differ among populations within a community, and the capacity of a community to eliminate health disparities is assessed by monitoring rates and trends in those areas in which differences are manifest. This section contains a discussion not only on the more commonly collected mortality and morbidity rates, but also on the behaviors that influence them, the risk factors associated with them, and the high-risk groups in which they are found. The categories chosen for organizing these data are not mutually exclusive—AIDS, for example, is both an infectious and chronic disease, and certain health behaviors, such as regular exercise, are equally cogent in school-aged children and adults.

The categories presented here reflect the *Healthy People 2010* focus areas and therefore are useful in assessing the health of a population in relation to national standards. Although addressed below as discrete areas, many health problems are interrelated and multidimensional, and interventions to ameliorate them often must involve biological, behavioral, and environmental factors. In fact, all of the 467 objectives in *Healthy People 2010* (USDHHS, 2001) cross-reference each other, confirming that problems in behavioral health often accompany disability, the infant mortality rate is influenced by income level and access to prenatal care, and sexually transmitted infections reflect modal behavioral patterns that characterize subpopulations, such as sex workers or adolescents.

Infectious Disease

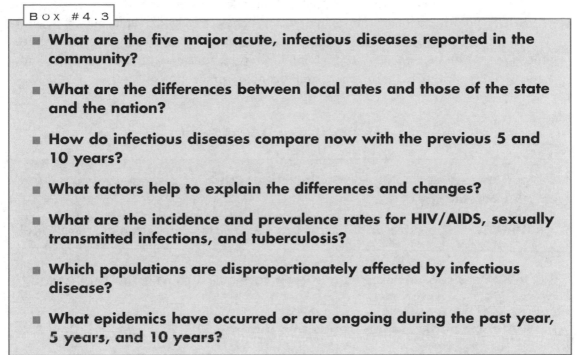

BOX #4.3

■ **What are the five major acute, infectious diseases reported in the community?**

■ **What are the differences between local rates and those of the state and the nation?**

■ **How do infectious diseases compare now with the previous 5 and 10 years?**

■ **What factors help to explain the differences and changes?**

■ **What are the incidence and prevalence rates for HIV/AIDS, sexually transmitted infections, and tuberculosis?**

■ **Which populations are disproportionately affected by infectious disease?**

■ **What epidemics have occurred or are ongoing during the past year, 5 years, and 10 years?**

Infectious or communicable diseases are monitored by the World Health Organization, the CDC, and state boards of health. Certain infectious diseases are mandated as reportable by federal and state law. These may vary among states and are modified as health problems change. For example, in the past, smallpox was reportable until it was eradicated as a public health problem. Some highly infectious diseases (measles or influenza), or diseases that derive from food or water contamination (salmonella or giardia), result in epidemics. An epidemic traditionally is defined as a greater number of cases than expected, found in a particular place at a particular point in time (MacMahon & Trichopoulos, 1999). This flexible definition allows public health authorities considerable latitude in responding to local-level situations. Tracking and controlling epidemics constitute a specialized endeavor, and epidemiologists usually are responsible for the initial recommendations for population intervention once their cause and location are determined. Community health nurses, however, may be the first to see these changes and are responsible for reporting them.

The infectious diseases most prevalent in the United States are influenza and pneumonia, and they disproportionately affect children and the elderly. Over the past two decades, both HIV/AIDS and other sexually transmitted infections have occurred at epidemic rates, with those under age 40, gay men, and IV drug abusers disproportionately affected. Most infectious diseases can be prevented through immunization, education, and/or screening and thus should be prioritized for primary and secondary prevention efforts.

Chronic Disease

BOX #4.4

- **What are the five major noninfectious, chronic diseases reported in the community?**

- **What are the differences between local rates and state and national levels?**

- **What are the differences between current rates and the previous 5 and 10 years?**

- **What accounts for the trends and differences?**

- **Which populations are disproportionately affected by chronic disease?**

Noninfectious and chronic diseases ordinarily are not reported at the community level until death occurs. There are, however, exceptions to this general rule. Many states and regions have cancer registries where prevalence, if not incidence, data are available. Voluntary health organizations, many of which are national in scope (American Heart Association, American Cancer Society) also are potential sources of morbidity data on noninfectious and chronic diseases such as cardiovascular disease, cancer, chronic pulmonary disease, diabetes, and neuromuscular disease. Coronary heart disease, cancer, diabetes, stroke, and chronic renal failure are the most prevalent chronic diseases in the United States (Brownson, Patrick, & Davis, 1993). Intervention at all three levels of prevention is indicated for chronic diseases. Since early signs and symptoms often are not recognized, and since health behaviors are related to the most common chronic diseases, primary and secondary prevention strategies are critical. With pharmaceutical discovery and technological innovation in healthcare, some diseases such as HIV/AIDS have become chronic as well as infectious diseases, suggesting new classifications and new ways of managing illness.

Chronic Disability

BOX #4.5

- **What is the rate of physically handicapped or disabled people in the population?**

- **What is the distribution by age and sex?**

- **How do these rates compare with state and national rates?**

- **How do they compare with the rates of the previous 5 and 10 years?**

- **What factors help to explain these trends and differences?**

- **Which populations are disproportionately affected by chronic disabilities?**

- **What percentage of the elderly over age 65 is considered to be the "frail elderly"?**

Closely linked to the prevalence of chronic disease is the rate of chronic disability in the community. Certain statistics regarding the disabled population are available from the decennial United States census. The increasing age of the American population and concomitant musculoskeletal conditions including arthritis, osteoporosis, and chronic back pain are the major causes of disability in the United States. Disabled individuals require routine health maintenance and secondary and tertiary prevention. While their conditions may not be reversed, their ability to function and their quality of life can be enhanced by community nurses through public action and policies authorizing parking, wheelchair ramps, curb access, public transportation access, special schools, and facilities. These interventions are a component of the public health infrastructure and just as important as clinical management in assuring quality of life, ability to function optimally, and productive social relations.

Behavioral Health

BOX #4.6

- **What are the mortality and morbidity rates pertaining to the following behavioral health problems?**
  - **Alzheimer's disease**
  - **Depression**
  - **Domestic violence (child and spouse)**
  - **Sexual abuse (incest and rape)**
  - **Suicide**

- **How do these rates compare with state and national levels?**

- **How do they compare with the rates of the previous 5 and 10 years?**

- **What factors help to explain any differences?**

- **What are the admission rates for addictive disorders treatment programs?**

- **What are the discharge rates for alcohol-related illnesses?**

- **Is homelessness a problem in the community?**

- **Which populations are disproportionately affected by behavioral health problems?**

Surveillance of a community's health status also includes the determination of various types of behavioral health problems. The burden of disability is profoundly underrecognized in this area (USDHHS, 2001), and data are essential for planning appropriate health services, whether ambulatory, residential, or inpatient, and for protective services for victims of abuse and crime. The suicide rate is an accurate indicator of the behavioral/mental health of any population; in 1998, it was 11.3 age-adjusted per 100,000 in the United States (USDHHS, 2001). The most prevalent behavioral health problems in the United States are depression and substance abuse, and these often co-occur, with 50 to 60% of the homeless suffering from psychiatric and addictive disorder co-morbidity (USDHHS, 2001). The prevention and recognition of behavioral health disorders, along with education to eliminate the associated social stigma, are necessary to address the pervasive impact they have on the health of all communities.

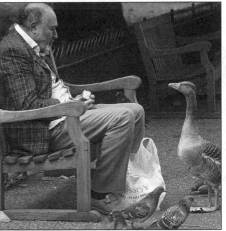

Photo by Daniel Althern, Solothurn, Switzerland.

Maternal-Child Health

BOX #4.7

- **What are the community's maternal-child health statistics?**
  - **Neonatal mortality rate?**
  - **Infant mortality rate?**
  - **Maternal mortality rate?**

- **How do these rates compare with the previous 5 and 10 years?**

- **What differences exist between local and national rates?**

- **How can these trends and differences be explained?**

- **What is the most common cause of death for preschoolers?**

- **What are the most common causes of morbidity in preschoolers?**

- **Which populations are disproportionately characterized by higher rates of morbidity and mortality, low birth weight and preterm births?**

Maternal-Child Health Behavior

BOX #4.8

- **What percentage of women in the district receive timely prenatal and postnatal care?**

- **What percentage of preschool-age children are immunized?**

- **What percentage of preschool-age children receive well-child care?**

- **What is the rate of teenage pregnancy?**

- **What is the nutritional status of mothers and preschoolers?**

- **What percentage of pregnant mothers smoke or abuse alcohol or other drugs?**

- **Which maternal-child populations are disproportionately characterized by detrimental health behaviors?**

Traditionally, some of the most commonly used health statistics focus on maternal-child health as a measure of the well-being of a population. Crude birth rates and mortality and morbidity data for mothers and children provide a rough, but meaningful, indication of the health status of a population. Most of the risk to infants occurs in the first weeks of life, and mortality rates for this period have implications for improvements in both the prenatal and postpartum environments. The successful outcome of pregnancy and the ability of an infant to survive through the toddler stage provide strong testimony to the health of a community and the availability and accessibility of maternal-child health services. Thus, they continue to be used as some of the most significant measures of public health of local, state, national, and international populations.

$$\text{CRUDE BIRTH RATE} = \frac{\text{Total number of live births}}{\text{Total population}} \times 1,000$$

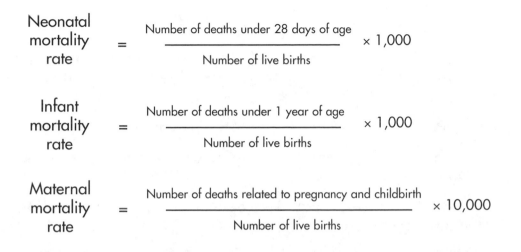

$$\text{Neonatal mortality rate} = \frac{\text{Number of deaths under 28 days of age}}{\text{Number of live births}} \times 1{,}000$$

$$\text{Infant mortality rate} = \frac{\text{Number of deaths under 1 year of age}}{\text{Number of live births}} \times 1{,}000$$

$$\text{Maternal mortality rate} = \frac{\text{Number of deaths related to pregnancy and childbirth}}{\text{Number of live births}} \times 10{,}000$$

It is important to remember that morbidity and mortality statistics are most effective in measuring the health of community when used in conjunction with other kinds of assessment data, such as health-linked behavior. In contrast to illness and disease indicators, health indicators may include, for example, the nutritional status of children as reflected in growth and development statistics, the completion rates of high school students, and the utilization of immunization services and well-child care. Federal guidelines recommend children be immunized by the age of 3 years for the following: diphtheria, pertussis and tetanus; measles, mumps and rubella; polio; varicella; hepatitis A; hepatitis B; pneumococcal pneumonia; and haemophilus influenzae type B. Maternal-child health is designated as one of 28 focus areas of the *Healthy People 2010* document. Significant emphasis is placed on behaviors that promote health, such as early prenatal care, breast-feeding, and smoking and substance abuse prevention (USDHHS, 2001).

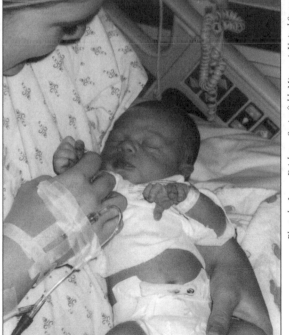

Photo by Jenny Erickson, Springfield, Missouri, United States.

School-Age Child Health

BOX #4.9

- **What are the leading causes of morbidity and mortality in school-age children?**

- **What is the nutritional status of the school-age population?**

- **What are the statistics on vision and hearing in the school-age child population?**

- **What is the growth and development status of the school-age population?**

- **What is the performance of the school-age population on national achievement tests?**

- **What proportion of the school-age population has been adequately immunized?**

- **What proportion of the school-age population receives routine well-child care?**

- **What proportion of the school-age population receives routine dental care?**

- **What proportion of the school-age population uses alcohol or drugs?**

- **Is violence a problem in the school-age population?**

- **Have there been any adolescent suicides in the past 5 years?**

- **Which populations are disproportionately characterized by high morbidity, mortality, or detrimental health behavior?**

The health status of the school-age population is measured not just as the absence of disease and disability, but as the capacity of a community to care for its dependent members. Combined with school-age-specific morbidity and mortality statistics, health behavior and developmental statistics permit greater accuracy in health-care planning for children's services and predicting potential health problems. The two most common causes of morbidity and mortality in children are unintentional injury (motor vehicle accidents, drowning, burns), and respiratory ailments. In addition, 12% of children under age 18 have a disability, resulting mostly from mental retardation and asthma (USDHHS, 2001).

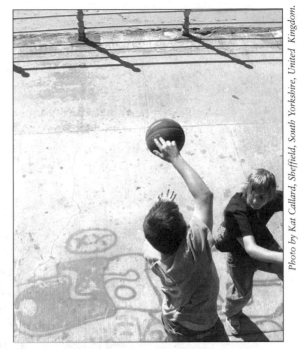

Photo by Kat Callard, Sheffield, South Yorkshire, United Kingdom.

Worker Health

BOX #4.10

- **What are the most common health problems found in the adult workforce?**

- **What is the rate of absenteeism in the adult workforce?**

- **What are the most common reasons cited for absenteeism?**

- **What percentage of the worker population has a routine physical examination?**

- **What percentage of the workforce engages in a routine exercise program?**

- **Which occupational groups are disproportionately characterized by health problems, absenteeism, and negative health behaviors?**

The health of our adult workforce is another measure of the ability of a population to meet the challenges of its environment. The development of health problems or a decrease in performance levels has serious implications for the economy of the community. Many causes of disability are related to the work itself and to working conditions: low back pain and carpal tunnel syndrome being two common examples. In addition, alcohol and drug-related problems, violence, and abuse often are identified and addressed in work settings that have comprehensive health programs. As ideal settings for primary prevention, the workplace is available for programs that address negative health behaviors and provide interventions to ameliorate them.

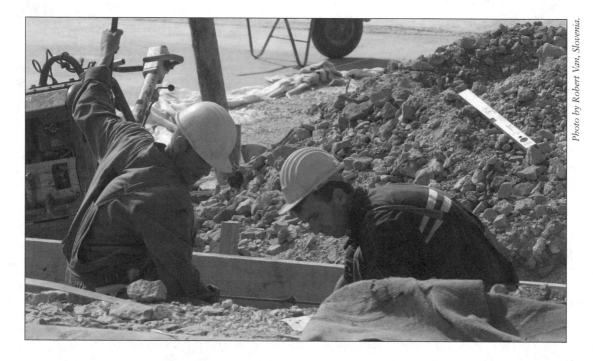

Photo by Robert Van, Slovenia.

Unhealthy Behaviors

Box #4.11

- **What percentage of the population exhibits the following detrimental health behaviors?**
  - **Tobacco smoking**
  - **Illicit drug use**
  - **Excessive alcohol use**
  - **Overeating or poor eating habits**

- **What percentage of the population exhibits the following detrimental health characteristics?**
  - **Hypertension**
  - **High blood cholesterol**
  - **Obesity**

- **Which populations disproportionately exhibit these behaviors?**

Negative health behaviors can be precursors to illness and often serve to place members of the population in an at-risk group. Accessing data on negative health behaviors is not easy. The CDC has standardized a survey, used by all states since 1994, that is reported in the Behavioral Risk Factor Surveillance System, with state-level data provided. Other sources of these data may include surveys by local organizations on smoking, substance use, and sexual behavior. Unhealthy behavior traditionally has been a target for nursing intervention and personal health services. Its usefulness in community health practice, however, lies

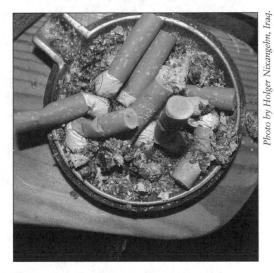

Photo by Holger Nixangehn, Iraq.

equally, if not more so, in identifying the disparities among populations and interpreting those disparities in health behavior vis-à-vis community determinants.

POPULATION HEALTH STATUS INDICATORS

The various dimensions of a population-based health assessment presented so far provide just a sampling of the unlimited range of criteria and tools that can be used to evaluate the health of a population directly. Special circumstances or problems may require more detailed information in one area of community health and less in others. It may be necessary to design yet another kind of assessment strategy specific to the community. It is always preferable, however, to make the best possible use of all existing data before creating a new instrument and collecting additional information.

Statistics and other health status indicators can provide powerful information about the relative health status of a population and convincing evidence about health disparities and the need to take public health action. There are, however, several caveats to remember in their use. Rates must be adjusted or standardized according to demographic characteristics and size of the community. Also, the morbidity and mortality rates in a small community may be deceptive when compared to a large community, and must be viewed over a longer time sequence to compensate for the small numbers. Most important, the data must be accurate and systematically collected. Death registry data generally are more reliable than data from birth registries, though one cannot always depend on the accuracy of the recorded cause of death. Certainly, not all births are registered and not all occurrences of a disease are reported—particularly for stigmatized health problems such as sexually transmitted infections, psychiatric problems, and alcohol abuse.

Although sources vary in the degree to which the information is accurate and reliable, dated or less-comprehensive information should not be discounted automatically. It may be the only information available. Using imperfect information simply requires that it be interpreted with caution for planning and implementation purposes.

The traditional starting point in assessing the health of a community is an understanding of the most commonly used statistical data related to the health of populations and environments, particularly when analyzed against the backdrop of cultural assessment data. Since judgments of poorer or better health status rely on comparisons with other communities, state and national statistics and indicators, and other time periods, a wide range of sources must be accessed. The 1990s witnessed a dramatic change with the availability on the Internet of health-related data. Many federal agencies that are sources of national health data sets list Internet links to state departments of health. **Table 6** lists Internet sites that provide not only comprehensive data, but also quick snapshots of health statistics at both national and state levels. Many of these sites derive from the Centers for Disease Control and Prevention, which houses the National Center for Health Statistics.

TABLE 6   INTERNET SOURCES FOR HEALTH STATISTICS

Here are some resources you might find helpful in your public health work. This is a mere sampling of the resources available. Please utilize your research skills and Web-search tactics to find more information on the area in which you are working or researching.

Web Resources	Description
International Health Resources	
http://www.who.int/en/	World Health Organization
www.icn.ch/	International Council of Nurses
www.unaids.org/en/default.asp	United Nations Programme on HIV/AIDS
http://www.aegis.com/	AIDS Information Global Information System
http://www.iarc.fr/	International Agency for Research on Cancer
http://icc.bcm.tmc.edu/	Intercultural Cancer Council
U.S. National and Governmental Health Resources	
http://www.healthypeople.gov/	Healthy People 2010
http://www.phf.org/index.htm	Public Health Foundation
http://www.apha.org/	American Public Health Association
http://healthyamericans.org/	Trust for America's Health
http://www.childstats.gov/	Forum on Child and Family Statistics
http://www.hhs.gov/	U.S. Department of Health & Human Services
http://www.os.dhhs.gov/	U.S. Department of Health & Human Services: listing of agencies and services
http://www.ahrq.gov/	Agency for Healthcare Research and Quality, U.S. Department of Health & Human Services
http://www.cdc.gov/	Centers for Disease Control and Prevention, U.S. Department of Health & Human Services
http://www.cms.hhs.gov/	Centers for Medicare and Medicaid Services, U.S. Department of Health & Human Services
http://www.cdc.gov/mmwr/	Morbidity and Mortality Weekly Report, Centers for Disease Control and Prevention, U.S. Department of Health & Human Services

continues

continued

Web Resources	Description
http://www.cdc.gov/ncidod/diseases/	National Center for Infectious Diseases, Centers for Disease Control and Prevention, U.S. Department of Health & Human Services
http://www.healthfinder.gov/	A service of the National Health Information Center of the U.S. Department of Health & Human Services
http://www.4woman.gov/napbc/	National Women's Health Information Center, U.S. Department of Health & Human Services
http://www.omhrc.gov/	Office of Minority Health, U.S. Department of Health & Human Services
http://www.cdc.gov/nchs/	National Center for Health Statistics, Centers for Disease Control and Prevention, U.S. Department of Health & Human Services
http://www.nih.gov/	National Institutes of Health, U.S. Department of Health & Human Services
http://www.cancer.gov/	National Cancer Institute, U.S. National Institutes of Health
http://www.ncbi.nlm.nih.gov/pubmed/	A service of the U.S. National Library of Medicine and National Institutes of Health
http://mass.gov/dph/	Commonwealth of Massachusetts Department of Public Health (Helping People Lead Healthy Lives in Healthy Communities)
http://www.census.gov/	U.S. Census Bureau
http://factfinder.census.gov/home/saff/	Basic fact finder for the U.S. Census Bureau main.html
http://www.whitehouse.gov/	U.S. White House
http://www.medicare.gov/	The official U.S. government site for people with Medicare
http://www.fda.gov/	U.S. Food and Drug Administration
http://www.cfsan.fda.gov/	U.S. Food and Drug Administration Center for Food Safety and Applied Nutrition

Web Resources	Description
http://www.conginst.org/	The Congressional Institute
http://www.nursingworld.org/gova/	American Nurses Association Government Affairs
http://www.consumer.gov/	Consumer resource
http://www.fema.gov	Federal Emergency Management Agency

U.S. State-Based Resources

http://www.health.state.mn.us/divs/chs/phn/resources.html	Minnesota Department of Health Population-Based Public Health Nursing Resources and Tools
http://www.asksphere.org/	Ask SPHERE (Southeast Public Health Educational Resource for Enhancement), a clearinghouse Web site published by the Southeast Public Health Training Center, which represents a partnership between academic and practice partners in Kentucky, North Carolina, South Carolina, Tennessee, Virginia and West Virginia.
http://www.pphtc.org/resources/onlineresources.htm	Pacific Public Health Training Center resource listing
http://www.bu.edu/publichealthworkforce/index.html	New England Alliance for Public Health Workforce Development

Environmental Resources

http://www.earthwatch.unep.net/	United Nations Environment Programme
http://www.wri.org/	World Resources Institute
http://www.panda.org/	World Wildlife Fund's Global Environmental Conservation Organization
http://www.scorecard.org/	The Pollution Information Site
http://www.lawvianet.com/	Environmental Law Net
http://www.epa.gov/	U.S. Environmental Protection Agency

continued

Web Resources	Description
http://www.epa.gov/enviro/html/qmr.html	U.S. Environmental Protection Agency Envirofacts Data Warehouse
http://www.epa.gov/ebtpages/water.html	U.S. Environmental Protection Agency, Water
http://www.epa.gov/oar/	U.S. Environmental Protection Agency Office of Air & Radiation
http://www.epa.gov/superfund/	U.S. Environmental Protection Agency, Superfund
http://www.epa.gov/oswer/riskassessment/index.htm	U.S. Environmental Protection Agency, Superfund, Waste and Cleanup Risk Assessment
http://www.isis.vt.edu/~fanjun/text/links.html	The Wonderful World of Insects

Population Resources

http://www.population.org/index.shtml	Population Communications International, Inc.
http://www.prb.org/	Population Reference Bureau
http://www.unfpa.org/index.htm	United Nations Population Fund
www.populationinstitute.org	The Population Institute

Topic-Specific Resources

What follows is a mere sampling of the topic-specific resources available. There are thousands of Web sites available to provide information and resources. Please utilize your research skills and Web-search tactics to find more information on the specific topic you are seeking.

http://www.cancer.org/docroot/home/index.asp	American Cancer Society
http://www.oncolink.upenn.edu/	Oncolink, Web cancer resource published by the Abramson Cancer Center of the University of Pennsylvania
http://www.acr.org/s_acr/index.asp	American College of Radiology
http://www.plasticsurgery.org/	American Society of Plastic Surgeons

Web Resources	Description
http://www.medscape.com/home	Medscape, from WebMD
http://www.natlbcc.org/	National Breast Cancer Coalition
www.komen.com	Susan G. Komen Breast Cancer Foundation
http://www.y-me.org/	Y-Me National Breast Cancer Organization

Health-Related Data

BOX #4.12

- **How can community-level data from the national census be obtained?**
- **How can data collected by the state health department be obtained locally?**
- **What diseases are reportable under state statute?**
- **What agencies are responsible for collecting and compiling local mortality and morbidity data?**
- **What is the unit of local data collection, e.g., town, county, district, etc.?**
- **What data relevant to quality of life are collected at local and state levels?**

THE UNITED STATES CENSUS

Mandated by the U.S. Constitution in 1790, the census is conducted every 10 years. Socio-demographic information, including various aspects of health and social life, are collected, analyzed, and reported for the entire United States and subdivided into states, counties, cities, towns, and census tracts. Conducting the national census is an enormous undertaking. Unfortunately, by the time the data are analyzed and reported, they are not current. The census is very useful, however, for showing trends over time and establishing a national database against which local statistics can be compared. The census data are extrapolated from a weighted sample that is representative. Some of the census statistics must be defined before interpretation; for example, the unemployment rate. The census also makes an important distinction between families and households, which is highly useful for community health purposes. Most of the census data are available on the

Internet and in libraries, and most states have a data bank center that produces a condensed summary of each geopolitical unit, i.e., town, city, county.

THE CENTERS FOR DISEASE CONTROL AND PREVENTION (CDC)

Located in Atlanta, GA, the mission of the CDC, an agency of the U.S. Department of Health and Human Services, is to promote health and quality of life by preventing and controlling disease, injury, and disability. The CDC is responsible for gathering information on all reportable diseases, collecting data from state health departments, and also conducting and sponsoring research on various health problems in the United States. In the *Morbidity and Mortality Weekly Report* (MMWR) published by the CDC, national information is summarized on common infectious diseases and news on specific outbreaks of diseases in various areas of the country. A most recent example is the CDC publication of the HIV/AIDS Surveillance Report. Similar data are available on the international level from the World Health Organization (WHO).

The National Health Survey, first conducted in 1956, contains synthesized information about the state of health and health services in the United States. Using probability sampling techniques, ongoing surveys of households permit estimates of the prevalence of specific health problems, including minor illnesses and disability. Since then, many surveys have been developed that constitute ongoing national data sets: for example, the National Health and Nutrition Examination Survey (NHANES), which measures the general health status of the total U.S. population; or HHANES, which measures the health status of Hispanic Americans (Idler & Angel, 1990; de la Torre, Friis, Hunter, & Garcia, 1996).

STATE HEALTH DEPARTMENTS

State health departments usually are a good source of relevant health data and reveal county-by-county differences in health status. They vary, however, in their requirements for reporting disease and the extent to which residents are surveyed for specific health problems. These data are particularly useful if health services are organized on a county basis. For example, in some states, records are kept on all firearms-related injuries treated in all emergency rooms. Other states may have the capacity to provide health status indicators to local communities. While most libraries have a government documents department to facilitate access to these statistics, increasingly these data are available through the Internet or through computer programs developed specifically for these purposes.

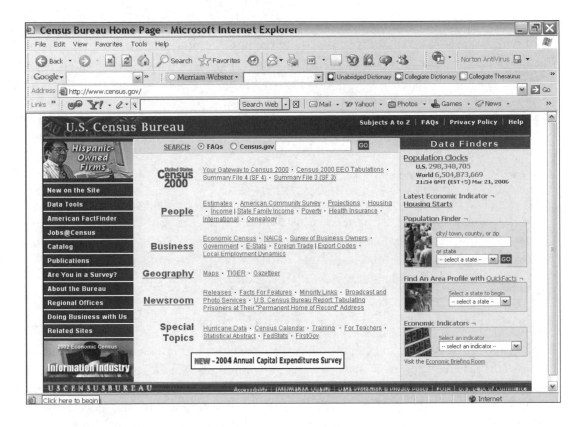

LOCAL SOURCES

Birth and death registries (which also are organized by the federal government) and state, municipal, and county records on mortality and morbidity statistics all are sources of current data. Schools and industry ordinarily keep records on absenteeism, accidents, injuries, and other health problems. Many record the results of personality inventories, intelligence tests, and various screening programs, as well as utilization data, such as immunization programs, counseling and education centers, and visits to the school nurse.

Records from hospitals, clinics, and other health agencies, including professional associations and healthcare voluntary associations, are yet another source of local information on health. Unlike school and industry records, they reflect only utilization data rather than health status data. They do not take into account all those who have a health problem (incidence and prevalence data), but only those who are receiving care. Since many people who are in need of healthcare do not access it for various reasons, utilization statistics fall short in accurately describing the level of morbidity and predicting the need for health services.

Information derived from all health provider agencies, therefore, must be supplemented with data from other sources to acquire the most comprehensive picture of the health status of a community. Local health departments may have data based on a recent assessment of health needs as a basis for local planning efforts, and thus are the repository of much useful information about the health problems of a community and resources available to deal with them. The county coroner's office can be helpful in gathering data on deaths by accident, suicide, and homicide.

HEALTH SURVEYS AND EPIDEMIOLOGICAL STUDIES

National, state, and local health surveys provide even more detailed and equally important sources of data about the occurrence, distribution, and causes of current health problems. Such surveys are undertaken routinely by the government, schools, hospitals, voluntary associations such as the American Cancer Society or American Heart Association, or universities engaged in epidemiological or health policy research.

ASSESSING THE HEALTH OF THE ENVIRONMENT

The cultural assessment in Chapter 3 identified topographical, meteorological, and climatic features of the environment that may place a community at risk for widespread health problems. The industrial revolution; urbanization; the invention of the automobile, telephone, and computers; and the development of nuclear technology have drastically altered the temporal and spatial dimensions of cultures throughout the world. The rapid changes over the past two centuries have intensified pollution and generated public health action.

Assuring the health of a community presupposes assuring the health of the environment with which its population interacts. Deviations from environmental standards for cleanliness and safety can precipitate serious health problems, as they affect the most essential requirements to sustain life—air, water, food, transportation, the workplace and dwellings. Indeed, the remarkable progress in the control of communicable diseases over the past century is a result not only of the development of vaccines and antibiotics, but also of the improvements in sanitation and a general rise in the standard of living (Allen & Hall, 1988; Gehlbach, 2005; Koop, 1995; Levy, 1998). Improving the quality of the environment also improves the health of residents and the social relationships among them. *Healthy People 2010* includes environmental health as one of its major focus areas (USDHHS, 2001).

The influence of the environment is not a new topic in public health (Armelagos, Brown, & Turner, 2005). Natural forces such as volcanoes, dust storms, weather depressions, floods, and insect pests have altered air, water, and food supplies in ways that have threatened human life. Over the centuries, humans have burned wood and charcoal, causing localized air pollution. The process of urbanization, however, has perhaps placed the environment at greatest risk. Pollution and cities go hand in hand, as large congregations of people strain the environment.

Urban life can result in overcrowding and environmental overload if sufficient resources are not available to meet the needs of a rapidly growing population. In addition to using, and sometimes exhausting, environmental resources, high-density populations often are associated with industrial activity that adulterates soil, water, and air with various forms of solid and gaseous contaminants. The aesthetic quality of the environment is an equally important component of a community health assessment. Foul odors, dirty streets or roads, unkempt housing, and unclean recreational areas—all give the impression of a disenfranchised population in which no one cares about the community where they live, work, and play. The effect is depressing and promotes a negativism that pervades the community. On the other hand, a beautiful environment that is uncluttered and pleasing to the senses is not only a signal, but also a source of community health.

Safeguarding the environment for the health of the public is an international problem, and even remote communities are affected by contamination sites located thousands of miles away. When the Chernobyl nuclear facility in the Ukraine experienced an explosion in its reactor unit in the 1980s, the areas at risk spanned all of Europe as well as parts of Asia. The U.S. Department of Energy predicted 28,000 excess deaths from cancer over this land mass, with other estimates ranging from 17,000 to 60,000 (Lichtenstein & Helfand, 1993). Thus, effective intervention for environmental health may require that community nurses work not just at the community level, but also in national and global arenas. International collaboration must be initiated to lower the levels of carbon dioxide emissions, manage the production and storage of nuclear waste, limit worldwide population growth to sustainable levels, and address the economic inequities that plague the world environment. These four factors are implicated in the self perpetuating cycle of ecological degradation found worldwide (Cortese & Armoudliant, 1991).

The environmental inventory in the following pages is, again, by no means exhaustive, but simply a guide to some of the most common environmental health problems faced by societies. It should be augmented or modified according to individual communities. The relevance of problems will vary from community to community. Industrialized societies, for example, will be concerned with nuclear contamination, while agricultural communities may be more concerned with soil contamination, insect control, and potable water.

Air Pollution

BOX #4.13

- **What is the quality of the air, and how is it measured?**

- **What are the actual and potential sources of air pollution?**

- **What contaminants have been identified as part of the air pollution problem?**

- **What topographical or climatic features interact with sources of air pollution to augment the problem?**

- **What local health problems are attributable to air pollution?**

- **What are the trends over the past 20 years regarding air pollution?**

- **How do these trends compare to state and national levels?**

- **Which populations are disproportionately affected by air pollution?**

The quality of the air is a major factor in promoting the health and survival of the human community. Unlike water, it is not yet possible to purify air just before it is inhaled. Exposure to air pollution contributes to a variety of health problems such as asthma, emphysema, lung cancer, and other chronic lung diseases. Although most health problems associated with air pollution are respiratory, eye irritation and dermatological reactions are also common.

Air pollution is a result of contamination of the atmosphere by airborne substances that are potentially harmful, not only to humans but also to animals and plants. For centuries, people have burned wood and its derivatives for cooking and for heat, thus emitting ash, smoke, soot, and dust into the air. It was during the industrial revolution, however, that contamination of the air received the greatest attention from public health officials, inspiring movements to regulate the burning of coal to control the amount of smoke and soot. Polluting "particulate matter" has expanded from the derivatives of wood to include aerosol droplets, insecticides, and herbicides. Cigarette smoking, traditionally considered a personal health problem, has now assumed significance as a public health problem, as research has confirmed the noxious components of tobacco smoke are damaging not only to those who smoke, but also to those who are exposed to tobacco smoking by others.

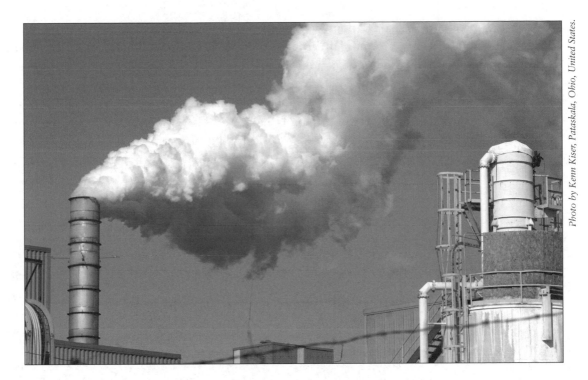

Photo by Kenn Kiser, Pataskala, Ohio, United States.

More than 50% of the population in the United States lives in communities where outdoor air pollution is a problem at some point during any year (Pope, Snyder, & Mood, 1995; Samet & Utell, 1991). The respiratory consequences of air pollution are mediated by the weather. Acid aerosols are worse in the winter in areas where coal-fired industry is common. Oxidates, including atmospheric ozone, are worse in the summer, especially midday to late afternoon, when the sun is hottest. Some of the illnesses related to air pollution include bronchitis, pneumonia, and the acute exacerbation of cardiopulmonary disease, asthma, and chronic obstructive pulmonary disease (COPD).

Today, the major sources of air pollution are emissions from motor vehicles, industry, and energy production. The emission of noxious gases such as carbon monoxide, carbon dioxide, and sulfur dioxide from petroleum and coal combustion and chlorofluorocarbons (CFCs) from propellant spray cans, solvents, and refrigerants, has contributed to contamination of the air. These gases are hypothesized to contribute to an intensified greenhouse effect by depleting ozone in the stratosphere, which provides a vital protective layer against lethal irradiation. If the predicted global warming resulting from the increase in greenhouse gases actually takes place, the consequences for health and human survival could be catastrophic (Leaf, 1989; McMichael, 2001).

While controversy remains about the timing and extent of global warming, there is little debate about its effect on rainfall, groundwater, food production, and ozone depletion. Topographical factors and climatic conditions interact with sources of air pollution to create even more pernicious and widespread problems. Mexico City, Denver, and Los Angeles, for example, have particularly serious problems because of topographical features that trap polluted air over the most populated areas. Communities that lie in a river valley often are subject to air inversion—that is, trapping of warm air on the ground by cooler air higher up, a common occurrence in valley ecologies. It is not unusual for the level of air pollution in such communities to be incompatible with national standards.

Water Pollution

BOX #4.14

- **What is the source of the public water supply?**

- **What methods, such as filtering or chemicals, are used to treat the water supply?**

- **What proportion of households use private water supplies?**

- **How frequently are water supplies inspected?**

- **Does local water meet federal standards for acceptable drinking water?**

- **Is the commercial water supply free from contamination?**

- **Have there been any unsatisfactory water reports over the past 5 years?**

- **Have there been episodes of outbreaks of disease due to water pollution over the past 5 years? Locate them on a community map.**

- **Is industrial or human waste being discharged into local water?**

- **Is the public water supply fluoridated?**

- **Which populations are disproportionately affected by water pollution?**

A safe and adequate water supply is essential to the health and survival of a population. From early times, water has been a vehicle for the disposal of various waste materials. Smaller communities may pollute rivers, streams, and lakes with sewage disposal and industrial byproducts. These bodies of water may then be the source of water for other communities further downstream. In most Western societies, the bacteriologic infections carried by water, such as cholera, have been greatly reduced or eliminated through water treatment processes, including the addition of chlorides. The pollution of both surface and groundwater by industrial waste, however, including radioactive materials and lethal chemical byproducts, is cause for great concern.

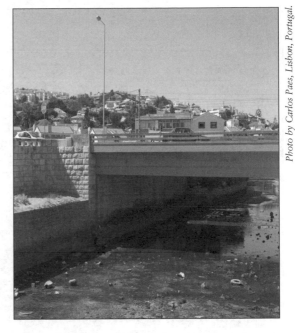

Photo by Carlos Paes, Lisbon, Portugal.

An environmental assessment must include information about the source of water and what measures are being taken to ensure its potability. This includes not only the public water supply, but also the water of those households with a private supply in the form of springs or wells. Clean water supplies also are important for recreation, such as swimming and boating, and commercial purposes, such as fishing. The health-promoting addition of chemicals to the public water supply has become a much debated public health issue in recent years—particularly with reference to fluorides. On the other hand, the possibility of dental health problems if the water supply is *not* fluoridated also is a public health problem. One of the *Healthy People 2010* recommendations is to increase the percentage of fluoride in the water (USDHHS, 2001). If, for example, large numbers of households do not use the public water supply, they should be identified as at-risk for dental health problems. Herbicides and pesticides used in agriculture also are potential pollutants, and water in such communities, as well as those bordering and downstream, should be tested specifically for these products.

Food Contamination

BOX #4.15

- Have there been any outbreaks or episodes of illness as a result of unsanitary or adulterated food products? How were they handled? Locate them on a map.

- What pesticides and herbicides are used to protect local food crops?

- Do local food products meet Food and Drug Administration (FDA) standards?

- Is food grown on or near sites where the water, soil, or air is known to be contaminated?

- Does the water used for irrigation of food crops meet safety standards?

- Which populations are disproportionately affected by food contamination?

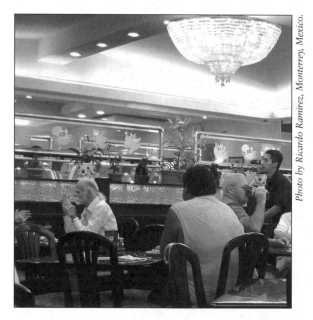

Photo by Ricardo Ramirez, Monterrey, Mexico.

The contamination of food can be caused by a variety of pollutants in the air, water, or soil. Dumping dangerous chemical waste products pollutes water and contaminates local fish products. The use of pesticides and herbicides is a threat to those who handle them, and downstream water supplies are especially toxic to young children. One widely used chemical pesticide—DDT—was so toxic it was banned in the early 1970s. In addition to chemical fertilizers, the purposeful addition of other non-food ingredients to enhance the flavor, augment the color, increase the size, and improve the shelf life of a product is another way man has disrupted the environment and precipitated health problems. Outbreaks of infection from food and milk contamination caused concern in the first part of this century, but concern has now shifted to problems created by the adulteration of food products.

WASTE MANAGEMENT

The ability to create a safe and healthful environment for a flourishing community requires the management of various forms of contaminants and other hazardous wastes, such as sewage, solid waste, chemical byproducts, and radioactive materials. Uncontrolled dumping of waste poses a serious threat to the air, water, and food necessary to support human life, not to mention the aesthetics necessary to enhance it.

Solid Waste

BOX #4.16

- **What are the sources of solid wastes?**

- **Where are solid wastes disposed of or recycled?**

- **Have there been any health problems within the past 5 years as a result of solid wastes? How were they handled?**

- **Is solid waste disposal in compliance with federal, state, and local regulations?**

- **Have any public recreational facilities such as parks, campgrounds, or beaches been condemned within the last 5 years as a result of solid waste dumping?**

- **How many breaches of sanitary codes have occurred in the last 5 years? Describe their geographic distribution in the community. How were they handled?**

- **Locate those areas in the community where the disposal of trash and garbage is a visible problem.**

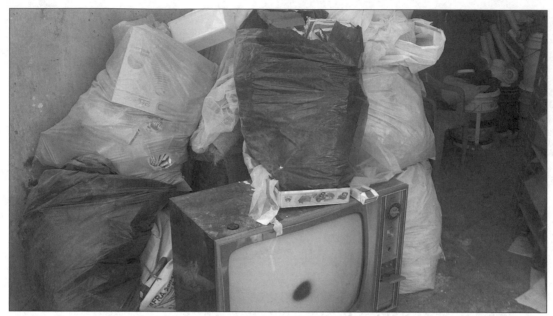

Photo by Jenny Solis, Atizapan, Mexico.

The dark side of postwar technology of disposable and nonbiodegradable materials can be found in the litter of bottles, cans, and plastic containers that pollute the land and seascapes. The collection and disposal of solid wastes and unwanted byproducts of industry are major public health problems, not only because of the potential contamination of water and food supplies, but also because of the unsightliness of the environment. Odoriferous and rat-infested dumps create both a health and aesthetic problem for community residents. As landfills reach capacity, financial and political controversies have emerged. It is not unusual for residents to oppose new plans for solid waste disposal sites. Illegal dumping has become a criminal activity, but often is outside the control of local public health authorities.

Sewage

BOX #4.17

- **What are the local methods for eliminating sewage?**

- **What are the local cultural practices and beliefs related to the elimination of fecal waste?**

- **What are the sources of sewage contamination in the environment?**

- **Is sewage management in compliance with local, state, and federal codes?**

- **Have there been any outbreaks of disease or other health problems within the last 5 years that can be attributed to problems in the management of sewage?**

- **What populations are disproportionately affected by sewage contamination?**

Every culture and community has firmly established patterns for the disposal of human wastes and the management of fecal materials. As with other forms of pollution, urbanization has created a problem by not providing the necessary facilities for adequate sewage disposal in densely populated settlements. Rural communities also require vigilance regarding the management of human waste. Septic tanks, leach fields, and cesspools are used in rural areas and need to be inspected regularly to assure surrounding water and land do not become contaminated. As with other forms of waste, the management of sewage has both health and aesthetic implications. Waterborne diseases such as giardia, cholera, and amoebiasis are the direct result of contamination by fecal material, either animal or human.

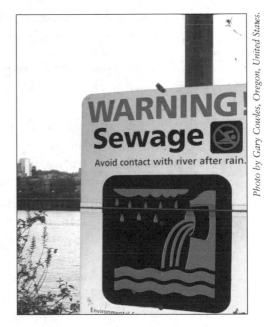

Photo by Gary Cowles, Oregon, United States.

WARNING!
Sewage
Avoid contact with river after rain.

Radioactive Waste

BOX #4.18

- **Is there any known radioactive contamination in the community? Locate the source and contaminated areas on a map.**

- **Has the community been a site for transport, storage, or disposal of radioactive materials?**

- **Does the potential for nuclear exposure accompany the economic base of the community?**

- **Is the management of radioactive materials in the community in compliance with federal and state regulations?**

- **Have there been any public health problems attributable to nuclear or radioactive exposure within the last 5 years? Locate them on a map.**

- **Does the community have a high rate of cancer, particularly leukemia, in comparison to state and national rates?**

- **Are there social or psychological problems in the community that are derived from nuclear exposure?**

- **Which populations are disproportionately exposed to radiation?**

While there are literally millions of contaminants that in certain quantities can be damaging to the health of a population, radioactive substances probably have received the most attention in recent years, particularly as the need for energy increases. Everyone is exposed to some form of radiation simply through natural exposure to the cosmic rays of the sun and substances of the earth. More dangerous levels of exposure come from medical X-rays, uranium mining and processing, nuclear power plants, and nuclear weapons development. The production, transportation, storage, and disposal of radioactive materials, such as nuclear fuel, present a significant health and safety hazard. Furthermore, the contamination of groundwater supplies can spread the danger far beyond the local community. Since the development of the nuclear weapons industry after the end of World War II, radioactive materials have been released into our environment (Lichtenstein & Helfand, 1993).

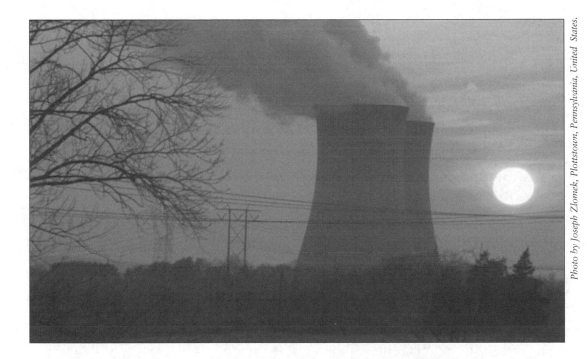

Photo by Joseph Zlomek, Plottstown, Pennsylvania, United States.

   The disposal of nuclear waste, given the long half-life of many of its toxic products, is of foremost concern. Various states have raised objections in Congress to the mass transfer of nuclear waste to be stored within their borders. As with other forms of waste, illegal dumping of nuclear material places the public at risk in spite of government regulation. The potential for sabotage and accidents in the storage and transport of nuclear materials poses both a physiological and psychological threat. There are many health risks associated with exposure to radiation, including leukemia and other forms of cancer, genetic mutations, and fetal damage. Careful records reporting the incidence of such diseases and health problems from year to year provide an important clue to the possibility of radio-active contamination.

Chemical Waste

BOX #4.19

- **What are the sources of chemical waste in the community? Locate them on a map.**

- **Are there areas of chemical waste contamination in the community? Locate them on a map.**

- **How does exposure to chemical waste relate to the economic base of the community?**

- **Is the management of chemical waste in compliance with federal and state guidelines?**

- **Is there reason to suspect uncontrolled or illegal dumping?**

- **Have there been any health problems or outbreaks of disease within the past 5 years that could be attributed to chemical waste?**

- **Are there social or psychological problems in the community that could be attributed to exposure to chemical waste?**

- **Has any area in the community been designated as a Superfund Site?**

- **Where is the nearest Superfund Site in relation to the community?**

- **Which populations are disproportionately exposed to chemical pollutants?**

Though not a new problem, the pollution of the environment through the disposal of dangerous chemical waste first received serious public attention with the Love Canal incident. In this case, hazardous chemicals were leaching from an abandoned disposal site located in an old canal where an elementary school had been built. Since the disposal began in the 1940s and was decades old, most residents of this newly thriving community in upstate New York were unaware of the disposal site where their homes were built. After moving into their homes, the chemical pollution traveled through underground waterways into yards and basements, as well as being vaporized into the air. Subsequent to extensive media attention and political involvement, studies were conducted that revealed an excessive miscarriage rate, although other health risks were not so definitively implicated. Many people moved their families from this site, and many more became aware of the difficulty of addressing suspected environmental problems through normal channels (Colten, 1996; Fowlkes & Miller, 1982; Levine, 1982; Newton & Smith, 2004).

Similar problems were encountered with Agent Orange, a defoliant used in the Vietnam War. More recently, exposure to chemical warfare agents in Iraq during Desert Storm was suspected of causing health problems, and the press even dubbed this the "Gulf War Syndrome." The uncontrolled dumping of the past century and the illegal dumping of more recent years continue to pose major health problems for the nation. The National

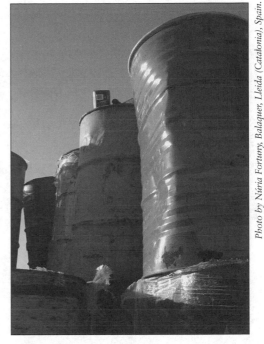

Photo by Núria Fortuny, Balaguer, Lleida (Catalonia), Spain.

Priorities List, also known as the Superfund Sites, scores hazardous waste sites by a hazard ranking system. There are more than 1,400 Superfund Sites in the United States, and the Agency for Toxic Substances and Disease Registry (ATSDR) assesses their potential for health effects. This federal program, designed to clean up huge sites of chemical, nuclear, and industrial waste, was established by Congress in 1980. Superfund Sites are designated by the Environmental Protection Agency (EPA), and knowledge of their locations is an important aspect of any environmental assessment (Neufer, 1994).

Each day, new research findings suggest exposure to dangerous chemicals is the etiology of many health problems, including various forms of cancer, birth defects, neurological disorders, reproductive problems, immunological disturbances, gastrointestinal problems, dermatological diseases, and vision problems (Salazar, 2000). According to Landrigan (1992), only 20% of the approximately 60,000 industrial chemicals used in this country have been tested for their toxic potential to human health. Sources of exposure include water contamination, lawn fertilizers, contaminated food and dairy products, pesticides and herbicides, and some disinfectants. The exposure of pregnant and lactating women, infants, and young children to these products is thought to be correlated to birth defects and blood dyscrasias, including leukemia.

Noise Pollution

BOX #4.20

- **Identify the sources of noise pollution. Locate the areas of greatest noise pollution on a map.**

- **What health problems are attributable to noise pollution? How are they handled?**

- **Are the regulations related to the control of noise enforced?**

- **Which populations are disproportionately exposed to noise pollution?**

Another often-overlooked public health problem is noise. Noise pollution is a byproduct of our advanced industrialization and technology. Although research in the area of noise pollution is comparatively new, it is now known to contribute not only to hearing loss, but also to stress reactions, irritability, cardiac disease, high blood pressure, and accidents. Community health nurses must educate the public regarding the potential damage of self-inflicted exposure to noise, such as power boating or loud music, and formulate and implement policies to control the amount of public noise created by aircraft, motor vehicles, and other noise pollutants.

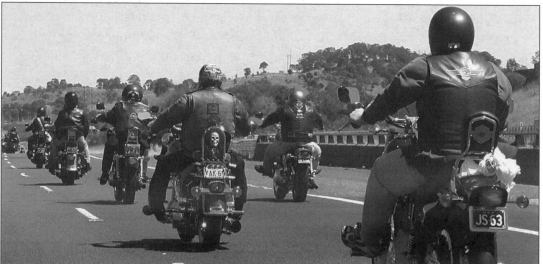

Photo by Neil Gould, Sydney, Australia.

Disease Vectors

BOX #4.21

- **Does the potential exist for vector-carried disease in the community? Locate the at-risk areas on a map.**

- **Have there been any outbreaks of reportable vector-carried diseases? How were they handled? Locate the areas on a map.**

- **Is there a problem with rat infestation? Locate the areas with the greatest problem. What has been done thus far to address the problem?**

- **Have there been any outbreaks of disease as a result of rat infestation?**

- **Is there a problem with insect infestation? Locate the areas with the greatest problem. What has been done thus far to address the problem?**

- **Which of the following insects pose widespread health threats to the community?**
  - **Mosquitoes**
  - **Houseflies**
  - **Roaches**
  - **Lice**
  - **Fleas**
  - **Ticks**
  - **Bedbugs**
  - **Biting flies**

- **What trends are evident in the area of vector infestation? How do they compare with state and national trends?**

- **Which populations are disproportionately affected by disease-carrying vectors?**

Although the emphasis in environmental health has shifted from food contamination and disease vectors to chemical, nuclear, and solid waste pollution, the control of insects and rodents continues to be a public health problem in many communities, both in the United States and internationally. It is well-known that many diseases are transmitted to human populations by rats and various kinds of insects. The role of the mosquito in spreading malaria, yellow fever, dengue fever, West Nile virus, and other infectious diseases is the major incentive for massive mosquito control programs in swampland areas. Cockroaches and houseflies are common offenders in transmitting gastrointestinal disease through the contamination of food. Insect vectors (agents) transmit disease by sucking the blood of the infected person or animal (host) and transmitting it to another person through deposits in food or through a bite.

The vehicle for control of vector-transmitted disease is entering the sequence of infection at some point to break the chain of infection among host, agent, and environment. This includes several methods, such as destroying the breeding grounds of insects (drainage of swampland and household sanitation), exterminating rats that harbor disease-carrying fleas, and using insecticides and physical barriers such as repellents, nets, or screens. The selection of method depends upon the life cycle and natural habitat of the vector and the host. Intervention must occur both at the community and household levels, including health education and inspection programs. In recent years, Lyme disease and other tick-born illnesses have received attention.

Disasters

BOX #4.22

- **Access the local and state disaster plan for the community.**
- **Identify potential disaster events for the community.**
- **Identify the cultural capital relative to disaster response in the community.**
- **Describe the disaster responses to recent emergencies identifying:**
  - **Local, state, and national involvement**
  - **Success of the disaster plan in preventing problems**
  - **Areas for improvement in local and state response capacity**

The Federal Emergency Management Agency (FEMA), now housed within the Department of Homeland Security, was established in 1979 with the charge of responding to emergencies that overwhelm local and state resources. As noted in Chapter 3, some communities are more at risk for disasters than others; flooding, hurricanes, tornadoes, and earthquakes can be predicted, expected, monitored, and prepared for in an organized fashion. While natural disasters may not be preventable, the level of community preparedness can significantly reduce the consequences. An increased empha-

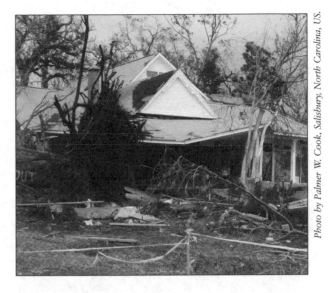

Photo by Palmer W. Cook, Salisbury, North Carolina, US.

sis on disaster preparedness has emerged recently as a response to the tsunami in Southeast Asia, the hurricane in Louisiana, and the earthquake in Pakistan, all occurring in 2005. Although not natural disasters, the Oklahoma City bombing in 1995, the World Trade Center terrorist attacks in 1992 and 2001, and the anthrax contamination in 2001 alerted the nation to a kind of vulnerability previously unimagined. These human-produced disasters are less predictable, and preventing and preparing for them is less straightforward. For example, FEMA designed a national plan to immunize all healthcare professionals against smallpox after 9/11 and the anthrax threat. One aspect of this plan was to recruit community health nurses as volunteers to National Disaster Medical System (NDMS) nurse response teams (NNRT) to implement this vaccination program. The plan, however, was never realized after various sectors questioned its wisdom and many individuals did not seek the vaccination.

All disasters have the potential to contaminate air and water; disseminate toxic bacteria in various ways; cause massive injury, death, and destruction; and induce pervasive fear, anger, and grief throughout communities. Thus local, state, and national disaster response plans are critical to safeguarding the environment, protecting the population's health, and instilling a sense of control and well-being in the face of overwhelming threat. Community health nurses are well-positioned to play a significant role in designing local disaster plans, as well as in building community capacity to put those plans into effect.

Crime

BOX #4.23

- **What are the 10 leading crimes in the community?**

- **What changes have occurred in the kinds and frequency of crimes over the last 10 years?**

- **Identify those parts of the community designated as high crime areas.**

- **What is the incidence of reported crimes against children?**

- **What is the incidence of reported crimes against the elderly?**

- **What populations are disproportionately affected by crime?**

In addition to clean air, water, and ground, an optimal environment includes housing, transportation, and community facilities that support the extension of healthy years and the elimination of health disparities. Casualties of this man-made environment include crime and accident victims suffering both physiological and psychological impairment. The safety and cleanliness of housing, workplaces, schools, streets, recreational areas, commercial centers, and other public areas also require vigilance and management, both to promote and protect the health of the public and to create an aesthetically pleasing context where a community can thrive. Moreover, a healthful man-made environment requires energy to provide the light and power to sustain health and improve the quality of life.

Personal injury crimes constitute a growing problem that has physical and psychological implications for the health of the public. Perhaps no other issue so dramatically illustrates the significance of the human environment in promoting the health and well-being of populations as personal injury crimes. Poverty, unemployment, the availability of firearms, drugs such as cocaine and methamphetamine, violence, victimization, racism, and sexism all have been correlated with the occurrence of personal injury crimes

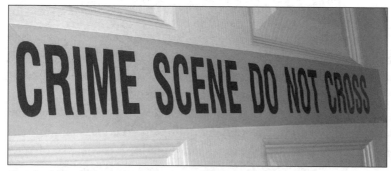

Photo by Shirley Harshenin, Winfield, British Columbia, Canada.

(Christoffel, 1994; DuRant, Cadenhead, Pendergrast, Slavens, & Linder, 1994; Hammett, Harmon, & Rhodes, 2002), as well as a more generalized fear of crime that inhibits healthy community interaction. The incidence of violent crimes against individuals, including murder, rape, robbery, and assault, varies among communities and populations. For some problems, such as domestic violence and incest, accurate statistics at the local level are very difficult to determine, and national statistics provide only estimations at the local level. Murder rates, on the other hand, are comparatively accurate. In the 1990s, firearm homicide was the leading cause of death for teenage African-American males (DuRant et al., 1994).

Problems such as these are new territory for public health practice, and there is much current research examining how to best ameliorate them. In addition to reducing related morbidity and mortality, *Healthy People 2010* goals include a 20% reduction in the percentage of homes where there are loaded and unlocked firearms (USDHHS, 2001). Public health efforts in relation to environments conducive to crime include identifying the risk factors and high-risk groups that are correlated with high crime rates. They also must include the identification of high-risk behaviors, such as aggression in elementary and junior high school students, and interventions to teach and model alternative means of conflict resolution.

In addition to having immediate and equal access to qualified protective services, all citizens of a community should have educational programs to help them avoid and report crimes and to rehabilitate victims of crime. The prison population in the United States tripled between 1975 and 1989 (Blumstein, Rivara, & Rosenfeld, 2000; Kellerman, 1994), and this reflects not only rising crime rates, but also the failure of jural-penal institutions, such as law enforcement and the courts, to respond effectively to this crisis. Some studies have found as high as 80% of prison inmates have substance abuse problems, yet many penal systems do not have rehabilitation programs in place. The proportion of the prison population that is HIV positive or has AIDS and tuberculosis is much higher than in the general population (Berkman, 1995; Hammett, Harmon, & Rhodes, 2002). The problem of crime and society's response to it has been the subject of much controversy—for example, gun control. Community health nurses have a pivotal role in prisons and schools, as well as the responsibility to inform politicians who establish policy related to crime, personal safety, and the penal system.

Accidents

> **BOX #4.24**
>
> ■ **What are the number and rate of the following types of accidents occurring in the community?**
>   - ■ **Motor vehicle**
>   - ■ **Poisoning**
>   - ■ **Drowning**
>   - ■ **Occupational**
>   - ■ **Falls**
>
> ■ **How do the rates compare with state and national levels?**
>
> ■ **What trends are evident over the past 10 years?**
>
> ■ **Which populations are disproportionately affected by accidents?**

Accidents continue to be a leading cause of death in the nation, disproportionately affecting young children, teenagers, and older adults. Motor vehicle accidents are the most common cause of childhood injury. Alcohol use is highly correlated with motor vehicle accidents, and this knowledge has inspired the now-common driver education programs in high schools, safe-driver programs for more experienced motorists, laws governing the number of drinks and acceptable blood alcohol levels, and the formation of the organization Mothers Against Drunk Driving (MADD).

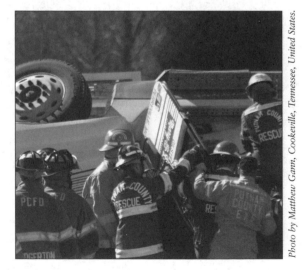

Photo by Matthew Gann, Cookeville, Tennessee, United States.

The rate of falls resulting in hip fracture in those over age 65 also constitutes a major public health problem, affecting women twice as much as men (USDHHS, 2001). Efforts to assure prompt attention to accident victims, such as volunteer first aid training, an emergency medical technician program, and adequate emergency transport, minimize the damage as much as possible.

The formulation of public policy and governmental regulation that will prevent accidents is equally as important. Proper labeling and packaging of poisonous substances, seat belt laws, and building regulations requiring window guards for young children are all examples of primary prevention policy. Making streets and highways safer for motorists and pedestrians, enforcing domestic and occupational safety codes to avoid accidents at home or in the workplace, and creating safe, protected recreational environments are essential activities in promoting the health of a population (Laraque, Barlow, Davidson, & Welborn, 1994).

Housing Construction

BOX #4.25

- **What is the general condition of housing?**

- **Does housing meet state and local regulations for safety, sanitation, and state of repair?**

- **What health risks are presented by the condition of local housing?**

- **What health problems, including accidents, fires, and outbreaks of diseases, can be attributed to poor housing? Locate them on a map.**

- **Which populations are disproportionately affected by substandard housing?**

In the cultural assessment of Chapter 3, the quantity, placement, and construction of housing in the community was addressed. In the community *health* assessment, sanitation and safety are the major concerns. Since people spend a major portion of their lives in households, the type and condition of housing—including living space, cooking facilities, and privacy—have a profound impact on the health of the population, including the growth and development of children and family interaction. Poor or inappropriately constructed housing may contribute to disease, crime, or safety problems such as high rates of fires, falls, and other accidents.

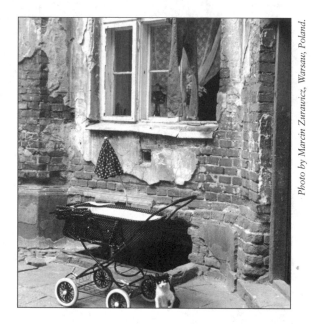

Photo by Marcin Zurawicz, Warsaw, Poland.

Improving the health of a community is highly dependent on the quality of the domiciles in which residents live. Community nurses are obligated to help residents recognize and address the potential hazards of existing housing and then advocate for them at the policy level to raise the standard of housing in the community. In this regard, they must work closely with official agencies concerned with the provision of housing, whether public or private. The kinds of problems encountered in community health practice include lead paint in older housing, radon gas in home basements, neglected housing repairs by landlords, and safety hazards in the homes of the elderly, as well as young families.

Community Buildings

BOX #4.26

- **Do community buildings conform to local regulations?**

- **Are codes governing the number of people and activities permitted in each building enforced?**

- **Are nonsmoking rules enforced?**

- **Do local employers conform to federal standards (OSHA) for occupational safety and health?**

- **What accidents or outbreaks of disease were attributable to breaches of health and safety standards in the workplace or other public buildings? What action was taken?**

- **Locate the buildings in which health and safety problems exist on a map.**

Like the private space of the home, the public space of the school, workplace, and other community buildings also must have a clean, safe, and acoustically and aesthetically pleasing inner environment. Most communities have codes regulating the capacity of buildings in terms of the number of people who can be there at any one time; the activities that can or cannot take place; the kind and quality of construction or renovation; and the health and safety factors of furnishings and installations such as plumbing, insulation, carpeting, paint, and wall covering.

These regulations on the interior environment are for the protection of the public, and breaches of the code require appropriate action. Code violations might include poor lighting, sanitation violations in restrooms, nonenforcement of smoking regulations, improper ventilation, or inadequate climate control.

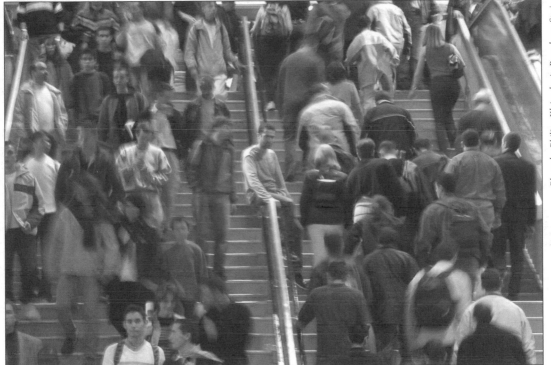

Photo by Philipp Kleinschmit, Barcelona, Spain.

The workplace is one of the most significant public interiors. The majority of the adult workforce spends at least 8 hours a day on the job, where they may be exposed to a variety of health hazards ranging from noise to dangerous chemicals to machinery. Similar to protecting and monitoring the natural environment, solving the problems of the workplace environment is complicated by the economic pressures facing many smaller industries, as well as their employees. Even when workers are at risk for serious health problems as a result of some workplace feature, they may be reluctant to take unified action if they believe their livelihood will be threatened. Although the protection of workers' health is ultimately in the best interest of the company, employers may be reluctant or even unable to expend the necessary resources. Establishment of the Occupational Safety and Health Administration (OSHA), an agency in the Department of Labor, was intended to protect workers in such situations.

Energy Management

BOX #4.27

- **What sources of energy—such as electricity, gas, oil, and kerosene—are used in the community?**

- **What is the major public source of energy?**

- **What private sources of power exist in the community?**

- **Is the source of public power adequate to meet the energy needs of the community?**

- **Is there evidence of wasted energy?**

- **What health or safety problems have derived from the type of energy source or its adequacy in meeting community needs?**

Urbanization, industrialization, and advanced technology require large amounts of energy to create an environment appropriate to the welfare and development of human populations. The conservation of energy is a public health problem that requires community-wide education and governmental regulation. In addition to the dangers of nuclear energy already cited, power dams pose the threat of floods, and electricity poses the threat of electrocution and electrical fires. The increasing use of wood stoves and kerosene heaters to reduce costly fuel bills also poses the threat of pollution and fire. Both domestic and public management of fuel and energy resources require an educated public and enforcement of safety regulations when using these resources.

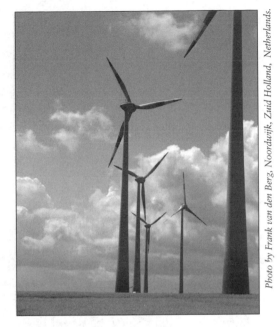

Photo by Frank van den Berg, Noordwijk, Zuid Holland, Netherlands.

OVERVIEW

This section contained a review of some of the major environmental problems faced by communities in rural and urban environments. The extent to which the environment can be protected from the pollution and contamination that accompany global urbanization is directly related to the sustainability of communities and the success future populations will achieve in obtaining optimum health and welfare. It is clear that for decades, very little thought was given to the environment. Society currently is paying the price with incidents such as the Love Canal. In a more optimistic vein, however, while advanced technology has contributed to the problem of environmental pollution, it is equally likely to reduce or eliminate pollution. Community practice nurses have an important responsibility to sensitize society to the potential hazards of a contaminated environment and to mobilize community support to fix it.

Legislation, policy, and economic sanctions are the major tools health workers use to combat environmental problems. Thus, emission standards for motor vehicles, regulations on dumping chemical wastes, and bottle recycling laws will have a greater impact on improving the quality of the environment and reducing the presence of disease, disability, and injuries than any one-to-one patient care intervention. Many environmental problems require even broader-scale, multicommunity action at the state or even national level. The movement of air and water, for example, carries contaminants across and through many communities, often far away from the origin of contamination and without reference to political boundaries. Effective control can seldom be sufficiently achieved by a local community. For this reason, the federal government has taken a major role in this dimension of public health. The EPA was established in 1970 to coordinate all activities that concern the quality of the environment: the atmosphere, land, and water. It has authority over the states and is responsible for conducting research, providing information, establishing and enforcing standards, and monitoring the quality of the environment.

OSHA was established to develop standards and coordinate safety and health oversight in the workplace. This federal agency regulates policy with regard to tuberculosis control in hospitals and is particularly important for nurses, who are one of the groups most affected by occupationally induced illness. The National Institute for Occupational Safety and Health (NIOSH), housed at the CDC, conducts research on environmental health hazards and recommends federal standards for OSHA and for mine safety. The Agency for Toxic Substances and Disease Registry (ATSDR) was created in 1980. While part of the Department of Health and Human Services, ATSDR is housed at the CDC and has a comprehensive mission with regard to preventing exposure to hazardous substances. These agencies all have comprehensive Web sites, and two other sites that are relevant to the environment are Toxnet (http://toxnet.nlm.nih.gov/) and the Toxic Release Inventory (TRI) (http://www.epa.gov/tri).

ASSESSING THE INFRASTRUCTURE FOR PREVENTION AND HEALTH PROMOTION

As a discipline, public health has endorsed prevention and health promotion as its principal methods of achieving health. Therefore, a community health assessment includes the prevention infrastructure as a fundamental aspect of the cultural capital of the community. There are three levels of prevention: *primary, secondary*, and *tertiary*, each of which corresponds to (a) the promotion of health at various levels of infirmity and (b) a set of health programs and personnel that make up the cultural capital for health promotion.

The goal of *primary prevention* is to reduce the occurrence of illness and disability and to increase health and well-being. Primary prevention strategies for a community's health presuppose a healthy population and ordinarily have included clean air and water, good sanitation, adequate nutrition, and safe environments for living and work. Today, many of our most intractable health problems—that is, those that grossly exceed national or international rates, such as low infant birth weight, homicide, and substance abuse— are strongly correlated with levels of poverty (Bird & Bauman, 1995; Blane, 1995; Blumstein, Rivara, & Rosenfeld, 2000; Reagan & Salsberry, 2005; DuRant et al., 1994; Roberts, 1997). It is an axiom of public health that as the standard of living of a population increases, so does its level of health (Evans & Stoddart, 1994). Thus, the effectiveness of primary prevention is measured by the quality of the physical and social environment as well as mortality (death) and morbidity (illness) statistics. Primary prevention projects could include river cleanup, nutritional education programs, and high school completion initiatives.

The goal of secondary prevention is to diagnose actual health problems as early as possible and restore a complete state of health in the shortest possible time. Building community capacity for secondary prevention is accomplished through screening for health risks and problems and timely intervention. Weight reduction, smoker cessation, and shelters for the homeless are examples of secondary prevention. Secondary prevention presupposes the ability to restore health. It is also measured by mortality and morbidity rates, but can be evaluated by such measures as response time of emergency teams, proportion of populations screened for specific health risks, and affordability and accessibility of health and social services. Police, firefighters, and shelters for victims of domestic violence are examples of cultural capital for secondary prevention.

The goal of tertiary prevention is to provide the best care and highest quality of life for those who are disabled or those who are chronically or terminally ill. The focus is on reducing complications, maintaining the highest level of functioning, and, in the case of terminal illness, making possible a peaceful and pain-free death. Hospitals, rehabilitation centers, and hospice care are examples of tertiary prevention. The effectiveness of tertiary prevention includes client satisfaction and restoration of function. The myriad community resources that support the goals of tertiary prevention were referenced extensively in Chapter 3—churches, governments that fund home care services, and voluntary organizations that donate needed medical equipment or provide support groups for the disabled and their families.

Although the goals of public health focus fundamentally on primary prevention and, in some cases, secondary prevention, all three levels make up the cultural capital useful for building community capacity. For example, health education programs for disaster readiness (primary prevention) may impact sufficiently on the results of a natural disaster, such as a hurricane, that will require secondary prevention and restorative activities and even tertiary prevention for injured populations. The integration of programs that support intervention at all three levels of prevention is ideal, not only for optimal outcomes, but also for cost-effectiveness.

Public Health Institutions

BOX #4.28

- **Describe the healthcare institutions that assume responsibility for monitoring and promoting the health of the public.**

- **What are the prevailing beliefs about public versus personal health in the community?**

- **Describe the healthcare policymaking arms of the community.**

- **What are the sources of financing for public health?**

- **What are the health facilities that make up the healthcare institution in the community?**

- **Who are the members of the community especially prepared to monitor the community's health and provide the necessary intervention?**

- **In what sense is the public health system controlled? Officers? Boards?**

- **To what extent are the healthcare facilities involved in planning for a healthy community?**

- **To what extent does the public health system take an active role in monitoring and reducing healthcare disparities?**

The cultural capital required for community health includes a special set of social institutions complete with beliefs and values, a group of personnel or "workforce," a network of facilities or agencies, and an organized set of functions or services. Although healthcare in the United States is considered to be highly developed, the limitations of its *public health system* are widely acknowledged (Allen & Hall, 1988). In *Healthy People 2010,* for example, it is suggested that the public health infrastructure in this nation is in a state of disarray (USDHHS, 2001). The changes that occurred during the 1990s in access to resources in the healthcare system have serious implications for vulnerable and at-risk populations (Estes, Harrington, & Davis, 1994). Without health insurance, many have no consistent provider of primary care and do not receive preventive services. Thus, they are at greater risk for more costly and even catastrophic health problems (USDHHS, 2001).

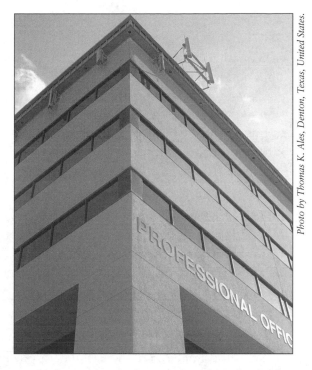

Photo by Thomas K. Ales, Denton, Texas, United States.

Not surprisingly, there is great variation among communities in the characteristics and breadth of their health infrastructures, i.e., the cultural capital dedicated to public health. Since communities differ with regard to their characteristics and problems, they will differ with regard to the personnel, facilities, and services needed to address those problems. But communities also vary with regard to the *resources obtainable* to address health problems. Indeed, one of the great ironies in public health practice is that the communities with the most problems usually have the fewest resources. As revealed in the preceding sections, these health disparities are detectable in both populations and environments.

A healthy community is a physical, economic, and social matrix that has the potential to extend the years and quality of healthy life and eliminate health disparities. Thus, the focus of the public health infrastructure is more on promoting economic stability, educational opportunity, robust community institutions, and universal citizen participation and less on the care of individuals. At the same time, there are many kinds of personal health services provided that qualify as public health interventions because they reduce risk or prevent widespread disease and disability. Such programs not only improve the health of the community, but also reduce the costs born by its citizens for expensive hospitalizations and medical care. Well-child care, flu immunization programs for healthcare workers, home safety installations for elders, school health services, prenatal clinics, hypertension monitoring, early detection screening for cancer, smoking cessation programs, and testing for HIV/AIDS are just a few examples. The consequences of not providing these kinds of primary and secondary prevention programs are grave enough to public health to have warranted their widespread administration.

In *Healthy People 2010,* there is not a major emphasis on institutions per se, but rather on the availability and quality of services. Within this emphasis, acute or tertiary care and specialty care are not considered priority areas; rather, the need has been identified in the areas of preventive care, primary care, emergency services, and long-term and rehabilitative services. Therefore, this assessment of community institutions attends closely to the provision of these services and care systems (USDHHS, 2001).

HEALTH DEPARTMENTS

In the United States, and increasingly throughout the world, the ownership of health institutions consists of a complex organization of proprietary (for profit), voluntary (nonprofit), and public or governmental agencies that, with their various facilities, personnel and services, make up an increasingly entrepreneurial healthcare system. Most incorporated or geopolitically designated communities—townships, municipalities, counties— have a health department as part of their government charters. Health departments are those organizations ordinarily provided by government statute to monitor and improve the health of the public and the environments in which they live. Typically, they are conterminous with geopolitical boundaries and thus organized in a pyramid of administrative accountability by town or city, county, state, and nation.

Health departments vary greatly in their range of responsibilities, but most include both population and environmental health services. Usually, they have responsibility for the bulk of primary prevention initiatives: public health education, communicable disease prevention, maternal-child health promotion, environmental protection, sanitation, inspection of food and health industries, emission standards, and the preparation of vital statistics, to name just a few. Depending on the community, they may be responsible for some secondary and tertiary prevention programs, such as control of communicable diseases, and direct-care services to underserved populations, even including chronic disease management. Monitoring health disparities increasingly has added to the ongoing responsibilities of health departments.

Traditionally, health departments were supported almost exclusively through state and local public funding from tax revenues and provided a limited range of services to residents at minimum or no charge. Now it is increasingly common to have at least part of the department's revenue based in fee-for-service activities charged to Medicare and Medicaid funds. The existence of health departments is a clear statement that health is a public responsibility. Unfortunately, because they are dependent on public funds, health departments are highly sensitive to the vagaries of partisan politics. Programs that receive full support in one party's term may be put on the back shelf as another takes office. In addition, when fiscal crises arise, public health programs may be sacrificed when they are not "entitlement" programs, such as Medicare or Medicaid.

Health departments generally are overseen by an appointed or elected *board of health*. It is not unusual for the majority of members of governing boards to have virtually no background in health science or healthcare. The possibilities for nurses to influence health as board members and as informed members of the community abound, particularly in the areas of assessment and program planning. Historically, health departments have been headed by physician medical officers. This has changed dramatically within the past few decades as community health nurses assume these leadership roles in public health, bringing their culture-based orientations. Local boards of health serve in the same capacity as trustees in the private health sector. The manner in which they are selected, their length of term, their roles in the wider community, and their philosophies on healthcare will strongly influence what the board of health can accomplish. One of the most important roles of the community health nurse is to educate politicians and official boards regarding the value of public health services for the sustainability of healthy communities and for reducing healthcare costs. Limiting expenditures for influenza immunizations, for example, will likely necessitate expensive hospitalization and medical care and increase the tax burden of the community. Similarly, the failure to support prenatal and postnatal care in high-risk populations results in greater public expenditure later on for special education and managing child health problems.

PERSONAL HEALTH SERVICES AND PUBLIC HEALTH

Although health departments are the centerpiece of the public health infrastructure, local hospitals, extended care facilities, private practices, and home health and ambulatory services such as clinics constitute a valuable resource for assuring the health of a community. Like schools, churches, factories, and recreational facilities, these health organizations constitute additional cultural capital that contributes to the public's health.

Hospitals, for example, ordinarily are viewed as providing secondary and tertiary services. On the other hand, hospital blood banks and disaster preparedness programs have helped to assure the community's readiness for adversity. Hospital records have provided important clues that can be used by epidemiologists to detect and explain various public health problems. More recently, hospitals are expanding their community responsibilities to play an important role in maintaining the health of uninsured populations through hot lines, ask a nurse health education programs, and health fairs. Emergency rooms have become 24-hour community health centers, and hospital-based cardiac health programs sponsored by hospitals help patients to limit their illnesses and extend the years and quality of healthy life. There are, of course, several reasons for this trend, not least of which is the encroaching competition from alternative health facilities, such as short-stay surgery centers or birthing centers, as well as from other hospitals.

Similarly, every community has different types and numbers of healthcare providers, most of which provide personal health services, but whose availability contributes to the public health infrastructure. Indeed, rather than recommending more and different practitioners, *Healthy People 2010* emphasized public health competencies that a broad spectrum of existing healthcare professionals should incorporate into their practices. These competencies include information technology, linguistic and cultural knowledge, biostatistics, epidemiology, environmental and occupational health, social and behavioral aspects of health and disease, and the inclusion of prevention in clinical practice (USDHHS, 2001). The report challenges educational institutions preparing a broad spectrum of entry-level professionals, such as nursing, public health, and medical schools, but also those providing continuing professional education.

To plan effectively for an appropriate healthcare workforce in a community, it is necessary to know what currently is available. Ultimately, the correct number and type of providers will depend on the number and type of health problems now and in the future. Demographic trends, however, have generated the need for health providers who are responsible for health promotion and maintenance and the management of chronic disease in children and elders. These primary care providers are expected to assure the coordination of care across settings in a cost-effective and high-quality manner, particularly in rural and underserved areas.

HEALTH PLANNING AGENCIES

In creating community capacity for public health, the agencies concerned with the coordination and planning of health and health services are highly relevant. Many kinds of organizations and types of ownership characterize a typical community health system. Growing in various directions, with duplication in some areas and great hollows in others, the entrepreneurial system does not lend itself easily to comprehensive, efficient coverage of the whole population. Federally mandated health-planning agencies have been established to assure that some pressing needs are not ignored, while others are not overserved. Planning agencies are responsible not only for coordinating and developing local health services, but also for the articulation of healthcare plans with other community plans, and for linking local health services to a wider network of specialized healthcare. Most communities have a formal body with the mandate to plan for the health of the population and environment. A challenge put forth by *Healthy People 2010* is to associate those agencies in such a way that health data systems can be organized into geographically integrated systems (USDHHS, 2001). One effort to systematize information and communication was realized with the adoption by most states of common health status indicators to provide a gauge of community health status.

HEALTHCARE FINANCING

In the highly entrepreneurial healthcare system that is likely to be found in U.S. communities, an assessment of financial resources is very revealing. There are many possible sources from which facilities derive their revenues, e.g., private insurers, public insurers, fee for service, charity, pre-paid healthcare plans, etc. Another approach to financing is to look at the financial resources that residents of the community have available to them, e.g., self-pay, health insurance, health maintenance organizations, charity—formal and informal— public assistance, or government insurance such as Medicaid and Medicare. In many communities, care of the medically indigent has fallen to the health department and public hospitals. Ultimately all services must be paid by someone. In assessing the public health infra-

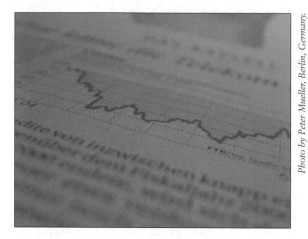

Photo by Peter Mueller, Berlin, Germany.

structure, it is important to identify health programs and activities that are publicly supported, i.e., without charge or at a nominal charge to qualified residents. These could include school physicals, dental hygiene, immunizations, and prenatal care provided by the health department, as well as those services provided by funds raised by voluntary associations or other community groups. The source and method of payment for health services will profoundly affect the distribution, quality, and range of services provided. Despite acclamation for the value of prevention and early detection, unless such activities are reimbursed or supported in some manner, they will continue to be omitted in the range of services provided to communities.

Beliefs About Public Health

BOX #4.29

- **What common beliefs are held by local populations about the cause, prevention, and treatment of public health problems?**

- **Are there local differences of opinion about what constitutes a healthy community?**

- **What public health interventions are a source of disagreement in the community?**

- **What age is considered to be a "natural" age at which to die?**

- **What differences in healthcare beliefs are present in this community?**

- **Do residents use more than one provider system?**

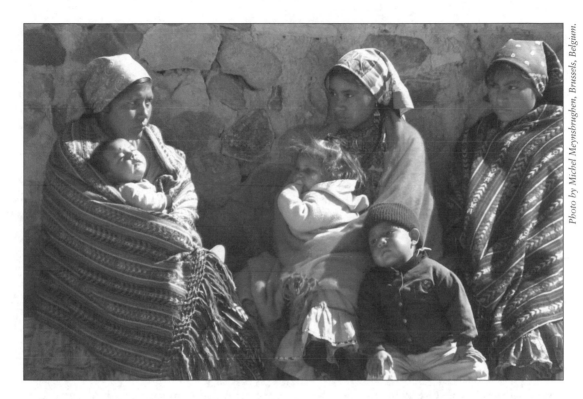

Photo by Michel Meynsbrughen, Brussels, Belgium.

While beliefs about health are not uniformly held or acted upon by all members of a society, it is nevertheless possible to identify a broad range of health ideas, values, and practices that guide and shape the public health infrastructure of a community. Almost all culture groups have theories of etiology or causation that influence behavior related to disease prevention and health promotion that are more or less embraced. In the United States, for example, the virus theory of infectious disease explains why individuals contract influenza, but it does not explain why some people acquire the disease and others do not, even though their exposure was the same. For this reason, the recommendations for immunization are not always followed.

The endorsement of public services requires, minimally, that people believe the potential for a public health problem exists, and that the problem is amenable to public health intervention. Some members of the community may view violence in schools as a singular, pathological event, rather than as an indication of widespread adolescent disenfranchisement. Others may view health disparities as just part of the natural order of society, rather than as a symptom of an unhealthy society. Even the most homogenous communities report a lack of agreement on what constitutes a public health problem and its resolution. Thus, the variation in meanings that specific social conditions and behaviors hold for different groups must be considered in planning for the public's health. A lack of understanding between health professionals and the lay public on the definition of a public health problem and the appropriate prevention and treatment can have a profound effect on the success of efforts to build community capacity and ameliorate the problem.

ALTERNATIVE HEALTH SYSTEMS

Finally, when assessing the public health infrastructure of a community, it would be inaccurate to assume that there is only one health system operative, and that people who do not avail themselves of the biomedical system are not receiving care. Rather than making assumptions, it is better simply to ask how people in the community protect their health. How do they make their community a healthier place? The answers to such questions can reveal the less-visible local healthcare institutions and the degree to which they are embedded in local culture and connected with other healthcare institutions.

Most populations pursue all the health resources available to them, and if, for instance, two distinct systems are in place, it is common for both to be used (Capps, 1994; Crandon de Malamud, 1994; Whitaker, 2003). Anthropologists have labeled this *medical pluralism*. Given the large populations of ethnically and/or racially diverse and immigrant groups in many communities, it is incumbent upon community practitioners to know the range of the healthcare infrastructure available in them. By far the greatest share of personal healthcare in any society takes place in the home, where methods of caring and remedies have passed through families over generations.

Most communities have institutions that are less visible, but provide the range of primary, secondary, and tertiary prevention in a well-organized, internally consistent system. Good examples are the *espiritismo* centers found in significant numbers in areas where Cuban and/or Puerto Rican populations reside (Garrison, 1977; Harwood, 1977a & 1977b). These centers usually are located in private homes, where services are provided in the context of group gatherings that have social as well as health functions. There are several reasons why it is important to acknowledge the presence of alternative health resources operative in any given community. First, much can be learned from these traditional modalities, such as the heavy reliance on group and community support as a vehicle for dealing with health problems (Alland, 1970). The power of group reinforcement, for example, is now being realized in the treatment of substance abuse, diabetes, cancer, obesity, and many other patient and family problems.

Second, the behavioral norms of subgroups in a community that, at first, may seem odd to outsiders, often are rooted in social or religious beliefs that have significant local importance in public health (Alland, 1970). Disregarding or disparaging them can be costly in terms of effectiveness in building community capacity. Third, by knowing the logic of alternative systems, it is possible to place scientific public health practice in a framework that may be more acceptable to community residents (Mahon, McFarlane, & Golden, 1991). For example, a program for expanding child health and prenatal care in a particular ethnic group must take into account norms regarding male and female role fulfillment, age-appropriate sexual behavior, and family structure, as well as the beliefs and practices associated with successful pregnancy and subsequent parenting. Not every client or patient will express the full range of cultural norms regarding pregnancy and childbirth. It is nonetheless important to understand and accept diverse beliefs and practices. Fourth, the leaders of such alternative systems are usually charismatic individuals whose local power can be tapped by community practitioners for social change.

SUMMARY

Like education, kinship, work, recreation, and other human endeavors, the pursuit of health has a set of specialized institutions, activities, roles, norms, and values in society. All societies have specialized personnel designated to care for the sick and dying (Alland, 1970; McElroy & Townsend, 2004), but also for promoting the health of people in communities. The health assessment of a community complements and completes the cultural assessment, and constitutes a powerful documentation of the strengths and needs that must be accessed and addressed in order to extend the years of healthy life and eliminate health disparities. Like the cultural assessment, it necessarily takes years to fully document and understand the health status of communities and their populations. These needs and strengths also are constantly changing; thus, the community health nurse's efforts in assessment must be ongoing and regularly updated.

REFERENCES

Alland, A., Jr. (1970) *Adaptation in cultural evolution: An approach to medical anthropology.* New York: Columbia University Press

Allen, J., & Hall, B. (1988). Challenging the focus on technology: A critique of the medical model in a changing health care system. *Advances in Nursing Science, 10*(3), 22-34.

Armelagos, G.J., Brown, P.J., & Turner, B. (2005). Evolutionary, historical and political economic perspectives on health and disease. *Social Science and Medicine, 61,* 755-765.

Berkman, A. (1995). Prison health: The breaking point. *American Journal of Public Health, 85*(12), 1616-1618.

Bird, S., & Bauman, K. (1995). The relationship between structural and health services variables and state level infant mortality in the United States. *American Journal of Public Health, 85*(1), 26-29.

Blane, D. (1995). Editorial: Social determinants of health—Socioeconomic status, social class, and ethnicity. *American Journal of Public Health, 85*(7), 903-904.

Blumstein, A., Rivara, R.P., & Rosenfeld, R. (2000). The rise and decline of homicide and why. *Annual Review of Public Health, 21,* 505-541.

Brownson, R., Patrick, L., & Davis, J.R. (Eds.). (1993). *Chronic disease epidemiology and control.* Washington, DC: American Public Health Association.

Capps, L.L. (1994) Change and continuity in the medical culture of the Hmong in Kansas City. *Medical Anthropology Quarterly, 8*(2), 161-179.

Christoffel, K. (1994). Editorial: Reducing violence—how do we proceed? *American Journal of Public Health, 84*(4), 539-540.

Colten, C. (1996). *The road to Love Canal: Managing industrial waster before EPA.* Austin, TX: University of Texas Press.

Cortese, A., & Armoudliant, A. (1991). Fostering ecological and human health. *The Physicians for Social Responsibility Quarterly, 1*(2), 77-85.

Crandon de Malamud, L. (1994). *From the fat of our souls.* Berkeley, CA: University of California Press.

Cuzick, J. (2003). Epidemiology of breast cancer—selected highlights. *Breast* (Scotland), *12*(6) 405-411.

de la Torre, A., Friis, R., Hunter, H.R., & Garcia, L. (1996). The health insurance status of US Latin women: A profile from the 1982-1984 HHANES. *American Journal of Public Health, 86*(4), 533-538.

DuRant, R.H., Cadenhead, C., Pendergrast, R.A., Slavens, G., & Linder, C.W. (1994). Factors associated with the use of violence among urban black adolescents. *American Journal of Public Health, 84*(4), 612-617.

Estes, C., Harrington, C., & Davis, S. (1994). The medical industrial complex. In C. Harrington & C. Estes (Eds.), *Health policy and nursing.* Boston: Jones & Bartlett.

Evans, R.G., & Stoddart, G.L. (1994). Producing health and consuming health care. In R.G. Evans, M.L. Borer, & T.R. Marmot (Eds.), *Why are some people healthy and others not?* New York: Aldine deGruyter.

Farmer, P. (1992). *AIDS and accusation: Haiti and the geography of blame.* Berkeley, CA: University of California Press.

Fowlkes, M., & Miller, P. (1982). *Love Canal: The social construction of disaster.* Washington, DC: Federal Emergency Management Agency.

Galanter, R.B. (1977). To the victim belong the flaws. *American Journal of Public Health, 87*(11), 1025-1026.

Garrison, V. (1977). The "Puerto Rican Syndrome" in psychiatry and espiritismo. In V. Crapanzano and V. Garrison (Eds.), *Case studies in spirit possession.* New York: John Wiley and Sons.

Gehlbach, S. (2005). *American plagues: Lessons from our battles with disease.* New York: McGraw Hill.

Glick-Schiller, N. (1992). What's wrong with this picture—the hegemonic construction of culture in AIDS research in the United States. *Medical Anthropology Quarterly, 6*(3), 237-254.

Hammett, T.M., Harmon, M.P., & Rhodes, W. (2002). The burden of infectious disease among inmates of and releases from U.S. correctional facilities, 1997. *American Journal of Public Health, 92*(11), 1789-1794.

Harwood, A. (1977a). Puerto Rican spiritism. *Culture, Medicine and Psychiatry, 1,* 69-95.

Harwood, A. (1977b). Puerto Rican spiritism. Part 2. *Culture, Medicine and Psychiatry, 1,* 135-153.

Howard, G., Anderson, R.T., Russell, G., Howard, V.J., & Burk, G.L. (2000). Race, socio-economic status, and cause-specific mortality. *Annals of Epidemiology, 10,* 214-223.

Idler, E., & Angel, R. (1990). Self-rated health and mortality in the NHANES-1 epidemiologic follow-up study. *American Journal of Public Health, 80*(4), 44-52.

Kellerman, A. (1994). Annotation: Firearm-related violence—what we don't know is killing us. *American Journal of Public Health, 84*(4), 541-542.

Kelsey, J. (1993). Breast cancer epidemiology: Summary and future directions. *Epidemiologic Reviews, 15*(1), 25663.

Koop, C.E. (1995). Editorial: A personal role in health care reform. *American Journal of Public Health, 85*(6), 759-760.

Landrigan, P. (1992). Commentary: Environmental disease—A preventable epidemic. *American Journal of Public Health, 82*(7), 941-943.

Laraque, D., Barlow, B., Davidson, L., & Welborn, C. (1994). The central Harlem playground injury prevention project: A model for change. *American Journal of Public Health, 84*(10), 1691-1692.

Leaf, A. (1989). Potential health effects of global climatic and environmental changes. *The New England Journal of Medicine, 321*(23), 1577-1583.

Levine, A. (1982). *Love Canal: Science, politics and people.* Lexington, MA: Lexington Books.

Levy, B.S. (1998). Creating the future of public health: Values, vision and leadership. *American Journal of Public Health, 88*(2), 188-192.

Lichtenstein, K., & Helfand, I. (1993). Radiation and health: Nuclear weapons and nuclear power. In E. Chevian (Ed.), *Critical condition.* Cambridge, MA: MIT Press.

MacMahon, B., & Trichopoulos, D. (1999). *Epidemiology: Principles and practice.* New York: Lippincott, Williams & Wilkins.

Mahon, J., McFarlane, J., & Golden, K. (1991). De Madres a Madres: A community partnership for health. *Public Health Nursing, 8*(1), 13-19.

McElroy, A., & Townsend, P. (2004). *Medical anthropology in ecological perspective.* New York: Westview Press.

McMichael, A.J. (2001). *Frontiers, environments and disease: Past patterns, uncertain futures.* Cambridge, UK: Cambridge University Press.

Morton, R.S., Hebel, J.R., & McCarter, R.J. (2001). A study guide to epidemiology and biostatistics (5th ed.). Gaithersburg, MD: Aspen.

Neufer, L. (1994). The role of the community health nurse in environmental health. *Public Health Nursing, 11*(3), 155-162.

Newton, L., & Smith, D. (2004). *Wake-up calls: Classic cases in business ethics.* Mason, OH: Thomson/South-Western.

Pope, A.M., Snyder, M.A., & Mood, L.H. (Eds.). (1995). *Nursing, health and the environment.* Washington, DC: National Academy Press.

Reagan, P.B., & Salsberry, P.J. (2005). Race and ethnic differences in determinants of pre-term birth in the USA: Broadening the social context. *Social Science and Medicine,* (60), 2217-2228.

Roberts, E.M. (1997). Neighborhood social environments and the distribution of low birth weight in Chicago. *American Journal of Public Health, 87*(4), 597-603.

Salazar, M.K. (2000). Environmental health: Responding to the call. *Public Health Nursing, 17*(2), 73-74.

Samet, J., & Utell, M. (1991). The environment and the lung: Changing perspectives. *Journal of the American Medical Association, 266*(5), 670-675.

Singh, G.K., & Yu, S.M. (1995). Infant mortality in the United States: Trends, differentials, and projections, 1950 through 2010. *American Journal of Public Health, 85*(7), 957-965.

Steenland, K., Hu, S., & Walker, J. (2004). All-cause and cause-specific mortality by socioeconomic status among employed persons in 27 U.S. states, 1984-1997. *American Journal of Public Health, 94*(6), 1037-1042.

U.S. Department of Health and Human Services. (2001). *Healthy people 2010.* McLean, VA: International Medical Publishing.

Valanis, B. (1999). *Epidemiology in nursing and health care.* Stamford, CT: Appleton & Lange.

Whitaker, E.D. (2003). The idea of health: History, medical pluralism, and the management of the body in Emilia-Romagna, Italy. *Medical Anthropology Quarterly, 17*(3), 348-375.

Woolf, S.H., Johnson, R.E., Fryer, G.E., Rust, G., & Satcher, D. (2004). The health impact of resolving racial disparities: An analysis of U.S. mortality data. *American Journal of Public Health, 94*(12), 2078-2081.

ACTION AND ADVOCACY IN COMMUNITY HEALTH PRACTICE

Healthy People 2010 identifies three major categories of community-level interventions for promoting health—educational, political, and environmental. Educational approaches include heightening community awareness, communication, and skill building. They include, for example, public messages to parents and teens about drinking and driving or social marketing projects on AIDS prevention. Political interventions comprise the public policies, laws, regulations, formal and informal rules, and understandings that guide individual and collective behavior. Policies designed to encourage healthful actions—such as seat belts and nutritional disclosure requirements on processed foods—fall under this category. Environmental strategies are measures that modify or control the legal, social, economic, and physical environment to be more supportive of health and well-being—for example, increasing the number of streetlights to discourage crime, encouraging physical activity, or improving the quality of air and water (USDHHS, 2001).

With only three kinds of interventions, it would appear advocating for community health is simply a matter of selecting, planning, and activating the most appropriate action for promoting health and resolving health problems. However, inspiring communities to take action that will assure a healthy future is not just formulating policies about the sale of cigarettes to minors or educating the public about the danger of obesity or cleaning up the environment. Moving from the identified initiatives (e.g., sex education, disaster preparedness, or simply creating a community health plan) into the cultural realities of community life, things start to get much more complicated. Mobilizing specific individuals and groups to plan a specific project to take specific action in a specific context at a specific time requires a solid knowledge of community culture. Communities are made up of people with diverse interests, goals, and values. While emergency room nurses may think motorcycle helmets are a good idea, riders may consider them an unnecessary violation of personal freedom. Some citizens, whose tax dollars support public education, may object to plans that include sex education in schools; still others may object to it not being part of the school health curriculum.

In Chapters 5 and 6, culturally grounded strategies for achieving the goals of *Healthy People 2010* are examined. The purpose is to explore the principles of organization and leadership that underlie successful strategies for community advocacy. Whatever the elusive nature of communities, the strategies identified in the following chapters suggest the effectiveness of community practice is related directly to (a) how well community cultural information is collected, organized, and applied, and (b) the power of the relationships between the nurse and members of the community.

REFERENCES

U.S. Department of Health and Human Services. (2001). *Healthy people 2010*. McLean, VA: International Medical Publishing.

CULTURE-BASED PLANNING FOR COMMUNITY HEALTH

Ultimately the goal is to build the capacity of communities to address their own health problems…better yet, to prevent such problems from occurring in the first place.

A community's capacity to increase the quality and years of healthy life and to eliminate health disparities requires continuous planning that is grounded in knowledge of its environment, population, and social organization. Community health plans must be fluid and flexible, responding to sociodemographic changes, shifting patterns of health and illness, and revolutionary advances in science and technology. This chapter contains an exploration of the foundation and process of culture-based health planning.

CHAPTER 5 OBJECTIVES

- Identify the value of health planning.
- Compare culture-based planning with resource-based and population-based planning.
- Outline the process of culture-based planning.
- Distinguish between an activity plan and a strategic plan.
- Trace historical and current trends in health planning.

THE VALUE OF COMMUNITY HEALTH PLANNING

Community health practice is necessarily future oriented. The health protection that communities have in place today is based, to a large extent, on the predictions and plans that were made 5, 10, or 20 years ago. What happens to our children, grandchildren, and the communities in which *they* will live depends on the predictions and plans made for 2020, 2030, and 2040. A thoughtful, informed design for the future helps communities to reduce the costs to society by effectively managing, rather than reacting to, change (Washington, 1998).

Take, for example, a Florida community that traditionally has been regarded as a retirement destination. Current population and trend data suggest, however, that the population is "greening," with young families moving into the area. A community assessment indicates that this trend, attributable to the local growth of techno-industry, is likely to accelerate. Without community planning, the programs supportive of young families and child development (e.g., education, recreation, child safety) may soon be insufficient to accommodate this restructured population. In addition to compromising the wholesomeness and safety of the environment for the children, unplanned change could disrupt community life and create competition between younger and older segments of the population.

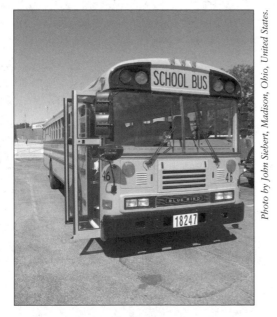

Photo by John Siebert, Madison, Ohio, United States.

Managing the future is both an ethical and operational imperative in community health nursing. Planning is a part of all nursing care, but it is so intrinsic to community practice that it is difficult to separate as a distinguishable phase or activity. In clinical practice, the familiar "care plans" outline the pathways to desired clinical outcomes. In community practice, the three core functions that promote healthy communities—assessment, policy development, and assurance activities (Quad Council of Community Health Nursing Organizations, 2003)—cannot be accomplished effectively without deliberate, continuous, and long-range strategies.

Accountable for the health of whole communities, and familiar with their residents and organizations, community nurses are especially well-positioned to lead the planning process. This is where, as culture workers and capacity builders, nurses bring citizens, problems, and solutions together in a plan for building a healthy community. The skillful integration of health programs with other community institutions such as schools, faith institutions, the justice system, and the workplace is central to assuring a sustainable, nurturing context for living. In health planning, the nursing profession has an unparalleled opportunity to activate its long-standing vision of promoting healthy people by creating healthy places (Ervin & Kuehnert, 1993; Ferretti, Verhey, & Isham, 1996; Gorosh, 1995; Washington, 1998; Salmon, 1993).

TRENDS IN HEALTH PLANNING

The *Healthy People* series provides a useful framework for the promotion of communities in which people live longer and have higher quality lives and in which disparities in health are eliminated. It is, however, one of only a few national initiatives in the US to explicitly address the complex relationship between healthy people and healthy places. Despite the original intention of health boards that first appeared in 19th-century England (Gehlbach, 2005), most health planning in this country has focused on the control of costs and the efficient distribution of health services, rather than on building and protecting healthy communities.

This health service orientation in planning reflects the widespread belief that healthcare is critical to the health of populations. Ironically, this contradicts a fundamental premise of public health science that such services are reactive rather than preventive: i.e., they respond to deviations from health, such as disease or injury. In this paradigm, health is defined as the absence of these maladies, which is completely inconsistent with the broadly endorsed World Health Organization definition of health as "a state of complete physical, mental, and social well-being and not merely the absence of disease or injury."

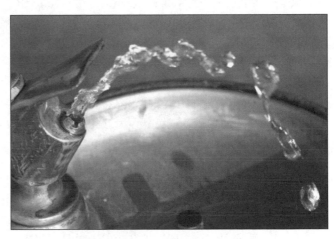

Photo by Ricky Gipson, Memphis, Tennessee, US.

This is not to trivialize the significance of personal health services and their profound impact on the individuals who are experiencing a disease or injury. The nurses, physicians, and other health professionals who provide care to those who need it deserve the admiration and respect they receive. It is clear, however, that major changes in the health status of whole populations and communities have occurred independently of the availability of medical intervention. In contrast, the impact of education; group support; satisfying workplaces; nourishing food; child protection; and clean air, clean water, and unpolluted land is profound, even though such factors are often viewed as external to the health system. The health of a population is a reflection of its relationship with the physical, social, and economic environment in which it is located. The failure in health planning to acknowledge the matrix of community life as a powerful determinant of the public's health is encapsulated in the distinction made by Evans and Stoddart (1994, p. 27) between "producing health" and "consuming health care."

RESOURCE-BASED PLANNING

In 1946, the federal government launched its first health planning initiative with the Hill-Burton Hospital Survey and Construction Act. This act provided funds to assist states with financing the costs of hospital construction. To be eligible for funds, states were expected to formulate a plan for the organization of hospitals and other facilities, based on the existing facilities and utilization data. In 1962, federal funding became available for statewide planning activities, and in 1966, the federal government demonstrated its commitment to comprehensive planning with Public Law 89-749, the Comprehensive Health Planning and Community Health Service Amendments, authorizing health planning on a state and regional basis.

Traditionally, health planning was centered in and on the health facilities and services themselves—the "bricks and mortar" of healthcare. Visiting nurse agencies, rehabilitation centers, hospitals, nursing homes, mental health services, and other kinds of facilities were established in relation to current demand and opportunity. This *resource-based* planning focused on utilization of existing healthcare institutions as a way of anticipating and organizing health services. Its underlying strategy was to adjust the existing services to the individuals and families who currently use them (McClain, 1978). For example, if a home health agency was used to capacity, more nursing staff would be employed; if a hospital pediatric unit was underutilized, it would be closed.

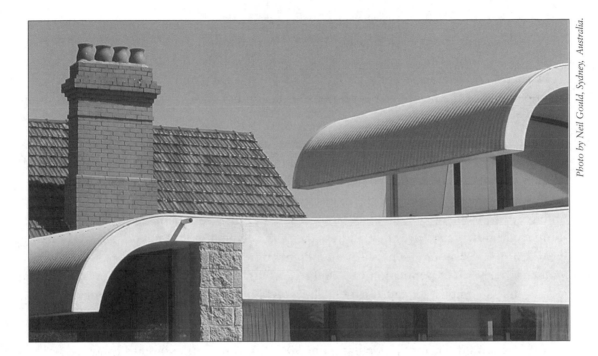

Photo by Neil Gould, Sydney, Australia.

Managing demand, of course, emphasizes the treatment of health problems rather than prevention of illness and promotion of health. Early health planning concentrated on the organization and delivery of personal health services with little regard for anticipating and guiding the development of activities that would promote healthy places and healthy people. Nor was there much of an effort to search for efficiencies, reduce disparities in access, control excesses, or manage the costly fragmentation and duplication of services. As health insurance became increasingly available to the general public (e.g., Medicare and Medicaid), personal health services became the almost exclusive focus of health planning. Third party payers (including state and federal governments) became, de facto, the contemporary health planners—usually in the form of gatekeeping.

To address the excessive cost and uncontrolled growth of health services, the National Health Planning Resources and Development Act (Public Law 93-641) established 205 local Health Systems Agencies (HSAs). Each HSA was accountable for planning the organization of health personnel, facilities, and services in designated health planning districts throughout the United States (U.S. Department of Health, Education, and Welfare, 1974). Responding to rapidly rising healthcare expenditures, its purpose was to correct the unequal distribution of services through regional planning and to control costs by reducing fragmentation and duplication of services. Each HSA was required to collect data and construct a health status profile (which, in most cases was a disease status profile). This area-wide profile then provided a basis for the formulation of a Five-Year Health Systems Plan and an Annual Implementation Plan. Applications for approval of proposals for new construction or alteration of health facilities were reviewed and evaluated by HSAs in relation to both the health status profile and the annual and 5-year plans to meet community needs.

In a valiant attempt to develop a "rational" plan for the distribution of health services, White (1973) developed a regional model for health planning in which he articulated resources and demands with populations and health needs. Although it does not deal with specific health problems, the model makes assumptions about the numbers and intensity of problems that are likely to occur in a given population. According to White, primary healthcare services that address the relatively common, but comparatively minor, health problems should be provided in a highly decentralized model and would serve a comparatively small population of 1,000 to 25,000. Secondary health facilities, including community hospitals, extended care facilities, rehabilitation services, and home healthcare, addressing problems of a more serious nature, would usually require a population of 25,000 to several hundred thousand to generate a definable demand. Finally, tertiary healthcare would warrant a population of 500,000 to several million to generate a predictable utilization to justify the presence of technologically sophisticated and costly services (White, 1973). In this plan, primary health is the pillar of a regional system. Quite rightly, White posited that the capacity to keep people informed, healthy, and comfortable lies in community-level services, where the impact of culture is most keenly felt.

Unfortunately, in the nationwide march toward allegedly "rational" healthcare, regionalization has been accompanied by a tendency to centralize secondary and even primary health services. With the advent of Medicare, size became a proxy for quality; traditional community health services, in which nurses worked with local institutions and knew all the residents and their families, were replaced with services from more centralized agencies.

In Massachusetts, for example, the advent of Medicare reimbursement for home nursing services signaled the elimination of "town nurses" that were supported with local tax revenues to oversee the health of town residents. Town nurses had a solid knowledge of the cultural capital in their communities. As long-standing "employees" of the town, they had great influence with residents and were aware of all the strengths and weaknesses of the community. They could enlist the assistance of community residents and institutions, identify environmental concerns, and engage local resources for promoting the health of the community. Persuaded, unfortunately, by centralized home health agencies, town officials saw Medicare as an opportunity to shift the cost of sick care from the town to federal and state governments. Unfortunately, it also eliminated the health promotion and disease prevention activities that the town nurses had provided in schools, the workplace, and other community institutions. It put community nursing (a primary service) under the control of centralized home nursing associations (a secondary service) with visiting nurses who often were unfamiliar with the local culture. In addition to affecting the health and well-being of community citizens, it ultimately was more costly (Dreher, 1984).

POPULATION-BASED PLANNING

In the 1960s and 1970s, epidemiological studies shifted attention away from health resources and toward health risks. This approach focused on existing and potential health problems in the whole population, not just in those who currently seek and use health services (patients). The population-based approach to health planning emphasizes health needs rather than health resources and looks at all the health problems and all the variables (risk factors) associated with those problems. Unlike resource-based planning, which emphasizes sick care, population-based planning strives to reduce risk and prevent illness and disability. The cost-containment strategy consists of primary prevention, health maintenance, early detection, and primary care.

Based squarely in the science of epidemiology, population-based planning has four basic steps. First, health problems are identified and the population is grouped according to distinct health needs, e.g., women, schoolchildren, elders, the homeless. Specific health problems for each group are identified and prioritized. Second, risk factors for each problem are identified through a review of the literature, and at-risk or target populations are determined. Third, the interventions needed to reduce or eliminate the problem are formulated. Depending on the nature and extent of the problem,

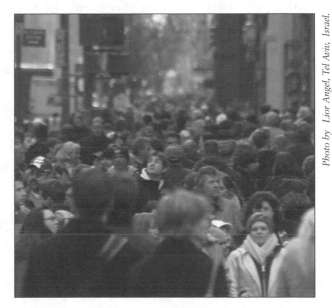

Photo by Lior Angel, Tel Aviv, Israel.

these could range from acute care to early detection to policy formulation. Fourth, the existing resources are compared with those needed to resolve the problem, and the gaps between needs and resources are designated as essential services that are incorporated in the community health plan.

Unlike resource-based planning, population-based planning initially ignores the existing resources and starts with health problems as they exist in the community, concentrating on what makes people unhealthy or vulnerable. Methods of resolving health problems are not limited to medical intervention or sick care but could include social marketing, policy development, environmental modification, and the development of public awareness. Population-based planning exposes the deficiencies and inequities in healthcare by drawing attention to those groups consistently at risk (pregnant women, smokers, the overweight) or underserved (the poor, underrepresented ethnic groups). For example, if hospital data and epidemiological evidence in an urban community revealed a steadily increasing rate of low birth-weight infants, the resource-based approach would be to expand the neonatal intensive care unit and employ a specialized staff to deal with this problem. The population-based approach, on the other hand, would first seek to understand the risk factors and risk groups associated with this problem. These could be economic, genetic, nutritional, occupational, or educational, and so on, and some or all of the risk factors could be characteristics of identifiable groups of people. Once the risk factors and risk groups are determined, planners formulate a strategy for risk reduction that might include, for example, family planning, prenatal counseling and monitoring, or nutrition programs.

By attending to unmet needs, instead of demand and utilization, population-based planning holds greater promise for prevention than for treatment of health problems. It is, nevertheless, a deficit model, focusing on the amelioration of specific health problems (smoking, STIs, influenza), usually by changing the behavior of individuals. In this model, these unhealthy behaviors become like diseases, amenable to treatment through personal health services. At the same time, many of these risks paradoxically are considered individual lifestyle *choices,* rather than problems embedded in the sociocultural matrix of community life. Fundamentally, the population-based approach assumes that the public's health will be achieved by addressing health problems of individuals, rather than by assisting vulnerable communities to build the capacity required to produce health.

Because of its problem-oriented approach, the population-based approach has the potential to divide community residents according to their allegiance to specific diseases or health difficulties. Pediatricians, parents, and teachers, for instance, will claim that services for children should be the highest priority because they represent the future of the community. On the other hand, cardiologists, their patients, and their patients' families will argue that cardiovascular disease is a leading cause of death, while geriatricians will cite the cost benefits of managing the care of older citizens. Of course, all are correct, but competing health problems and special interest health politics only serve to impede the development of a comprehensive community-based plan.

CULTURE-BASED PLANNING

Given the history and magnitude of state, regional, and national health planning, why is it that efforts to control cost have ended up costing more and producing less? Why is it that identified solutions do not produce the desired outcomes? And why is it that health disparities exist in a country so rich in resources? At least some of the answers to such questions lie, once again, in the disinclination of planners to take into account that murky, complex, sociocultural matrix. The failure of many resource-based and population-based plans can be traced to an exclusive concern with rational factors such as cost, time, and distance and a disregard for cultural factors, including local values, behavior, and institutions.

For example, the plan to close a small, religion-affiliated community hospital was considered rational because the hospital provided a limited number of services at a high

cost that were duplicated in a larger, better-equipped medical center nearby. The resources derived from closing the hospital were to be redirected to needed initiatives that could improve the health of the community. What the planners failed to realize, however, was that the old hospital had a long history of serving local residents and was a major community employer. As such, it gleaned both sentiment and support from community residents. The dominant ethnic/religious group in the community perceived this action as another threat and disrespect for its traditions. Champions for retaining the hospital also included labor unions, hospital employees, and powerful politicians working on behalf of their constituencies. To the citizens of this com-

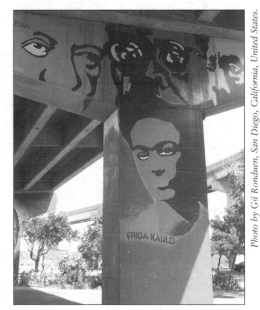

Photo by Gil Ronduen, San Diego, California, United States.

munity, the closing of the hospital was not just about rational healthcare. In fact, it really was not about healthcare at all. Rather, it was about community self-determination. It was about religion, politics, economics, and the social representation of community life.

This example is not intended to suggest that fiscal responsibility in health planning is not important. It does suggest, however, that planners may run into difficulty if consideration is not given to the cultural matrix of both the problem and solution. While popular sentiment and employment factors may be insufficient to maintain a costly facility, they must be given full consideration in the community health plans to discontinue the facility. In the example just presented, a culturally rational health plan might have included a strategy for dealing with the employment issues or a proposal for converting the hospital to another kind of health facility needed by the community. It might have included enlisting the community stakeholders, e.g., hospital workers, political leaders, and religious leaders early in the planning and perhaps arranging a ceremony that celebrated the hospital and its contribution to the community. Culture-based planning is an attempt to shift the emphasis in health planning from an almost exclusive concern with health services and health problems to include the production of health through the identification and deployment of cultural capital. Population-based planning identifies the risk factors and health problems in a population, but it does not inform planners of the best strategies to address them. Thus, even greatly needed initiatives for nutrition education, family planning, chemical-dependency prevention, or sanitation programs can be undone locally for reasons that have nothing to do with epidemiological evidence of need (Yakoob & Whiteford, 1994).

A culturally rational plan is one that makes sense to the people who live there. Plans for preventing and treating alcohol abuse in a community where the consumption of alcohol has both social and economic value will be different from one designed for a community in which the consumption of alcohol is regarded as deviant behavior. Plans to reduce the rate of adolescent pregnancy will be different in a community where parents place a high premium on chastity from one in which pregnancy is regarded as a normal and welcome event, signaling an adolescent girl's transition to womanhood. Likewise, programs for reducing the consumption of high cholesterol foods may not be particularly welcome in communities where meat production is the economic base.

Culture-based planning uses strategies from both resource-based and population-based planning, but expands the epidemiological, problem-oriented methods to action based on a cultural assessment and analysis of the local community. For example, in spite of our affluent society, obesity in children as well as adults constitutes a serious national problem. Many of the goals to address this issue, established in *Healthy People 2000*, have shown little or no progress. In fact, the proportion of self-identified overweight adults who report consuming fewer calories and exercising more, decreased from 1985 to 1995. More than ⅓ of American adults are now considered overweight, compared with 26% in the late 1970s. Ethnic disparities in obesity exist, and the increasing prevalence is not limited to adults. Morbidity associated with obesity, such diabetes, is observable in both sexes.

Using resource-based planning to address the burgeoning problem of obesity would require increased availability of products and services to accommodate the individuals seeking treatment. These might include opening more weight-loss clinics, developing weight-loss pharmaceutical products, educating more physicians and other providers to specialize in weight-loss management, and opening surgical centers focused on gastrointestinal bypass and plastic surgeries. Interestingly, all of these system interventions have occurred, with no impact on the growing national problem of obesity. Using population-based planning, additional solutions emerge, including social marketing; government regulations requiring the labeling of caloric, carbohydrate, and fat content on processed foods; more books on weight loss; and self-help groups—solutions that have been equally ineffective in stemming the rates of obesity.

But like countless other national health problems for which medical treatment and lifestyle changes are recommended (smoking, STIs), both the determinants and the solutions are most likely to be found in the cultural context of community life, e.g., how are dietary practices and food consumption related to work patterns, school menus, recreational activities, housing, communication, ethnicity, traditional celebrations, and the economy? Which community organizations, such as churches or schools, would be most effective in addressing obesity? It is at the community level that clinical, policy, educational, and environmental approaches can be combined in a multiple-strategy intervention to determine and address the multiple factors influencing diet and nutrition.

An understanding of local culture permits one to see how both problems and solutions are linked to other problems and solutions. The connections, for instance, among obesity in teenagers, poor dietary habits, low self-esteem, poor school performance, nonparticipation in sports and other extracurricular activities, failure to complete high school, unintended pregnancy, drug abuse, and a myriad of other problems are observable when placed against the backdrop of a community and its people, places, and institutions. Problems in the areas of health, education, occupation, housing, safety, and nutrition are all part of the same fundamental social and economic dislocations that create fragile communities and vulnerable populations.

It often is assumed that policies generated at the national level have a predictable outcome at the local level. The experience of many communities reveals, however, that the relationship between the suprastructure, where health planning and policymaking ordinarily take place, and the infrastructure, where plans and policies are executed, is not uniform and predictable. Like resource-based planning, population-based planning tends to be regional. Epidemiological data generally are collected at the supracommunity level and report the incidence and prevalence of health problems for large populations. Likewise, policy, regulation, public education, and social marketing are likely to be formulated and implemented at state and national levels, transcending specific communities. But it is at the community level where federal and state programs sink or swim, where citizens feel influence and exercise power, where resistance or support is most keenly experienced, and where the complex relationships between people and their environments are most reactive (Clinton, 1979). Those who have been involved in comprehensive health planning for some time can describe a pathway strewn with federal- and state-funded programs that either died in the process or were redirected at the community level, never fulfilling their intent (Hill, 1988).

COMMUNITY PARTICIPATION IN HEALTH PLANNING

The collaboration between community health professionals and lay citizens is a hallmark of community health practice. This is not a new concept in nursing; the principle that care plans are most successful when conceived in consultation with the patient and family has long been endorsed. Similarly, planning for the health of communities is most effective when conducted in collaboration with community members. The Hill-Burton Act of 1946 was the first formal attempt to include community representation in planning. It also opened health planning and policymaking to greater community participation by requiring citizen participation on all health planning boards. Subsequently, the Comprehensive Health Planning Act of 1966 encouraged strong citizen participation in community health planning efforts. Taking citizen participation even further, the Health Planning Act of 1974 mandated a citizen majority on health planning boards and was heralded as a major breakthrough for community-wide participation. Since 51% of the HSA boards had to be lay consumers, citizen participation on health-planning boards became a major vehicle for cultural competence. It was an expression of partnership in which the provider brought technical knowledge to the planning table, while citizens brought the community perspective. Community representatives, for example, might have seen a hospital not just as a health facility, but as an employer, a business, a vehicle for social mobility, a religiously sanctified place where their children were born or their parents died, or simply as a community tradition (Hornberger & Cobb, 1998).

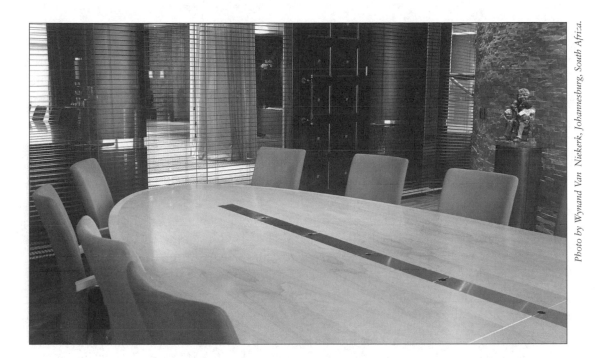

Photo by Wynand Van Niekerk, Johannesburg, South Africa.

Unfortunately, the experience of mandated citizen involvement led to some disillusionment over the role and function of citizens in health planning (Steckler & Herzog, 1979). Many provider groups and organizations elected to view the citizen majority as adversaries, rather than as partners in healthcare planning, and found effective ways to limit their contributions despite their numerical dominance. Even though their contributions were never intended to be in the area of technical knowledge, their lack of it seriously hampered their participation (Lassiter, 1992). Unprepared for their roles in evaluating proposals or suggesting sophisticated resolutions to health problems, citizen members often were co-opted to support provider objectives, particularly in the area of facilities planning. More troubling than the seduction of citizen representatives, however, were official health-planning policies in which communities were portrayed as culturally monolithic, where like-minded people sit down and, through consensus, reach similar conclusions about what needs to be done and how, when, and who should do it.

As we have discovered, however, a community's population does not have to be of one mind to be a community. Although planning goals are derived from an assessment of community needs, they are identified, modified, and prioritized by the availability of resources and competing community interests. It is, therefore, normal in health planning for goal setting and prioritization to be highly politicized processes, as various groups within the community compete for limited resources. The professional citizen-representatives of a community, who appear again and again on various community boards, are likely to be as self-interested as any other board member and as likely to disagree with other citizens as they are with health professionals. Representatives *from* the community are not necessarily representatives *of* the community (Bibeau, 1997).

Despite the somewhat disappointing results of mandated citizen participation, the nonprovider citizen continues to have a valuable role to play in community health planning, particularly in assuring that plans created in committee will be implemented in the community (Paine-Andrews, Francisco, & Fawcett, 1994; Satia, Mavalankar, & Sharma, 1994). It is a well-accepted premise of organized planning that those who will be involved in the implementation of a plan also should be involved in its formulation, and Davidge and Pearson (1995) recommend lay citizens should be part of the process right from the assessment phase. Community health planners should share national and state health-planning goals and guidelines with the citizenry and select representatives who are sufficiently influential to balance the views of providers with those of the community.

The health of a community is the shared responsibility of all its residents, families, and organizations. Culture-based planning requires local stakeholders to become invested in solving problems and promoting health. Because community health planning covers such a broad range of health services, it is impossible for every kind of provider and every sector of the community to be represented on every health-planning committee. But overall health planning should provide the opportunity for those directly concerned with a particular community health issue, both citizens and providers, to become actively involved through subcommittees, consultation, and public hearings. Most issues surrounding health, health disparities, and quality of life are sufficiently complex to warrant the participation of multiple sectors of the community—social, educational, religious, governmental, economic, recreational, and occupational. Continuing with the example of obesity among adolescents, stakeholders might include parents, teenagers, high school coaches, nurse-midwives, teachers, weight-reduction program staff, cardiologists, endocrinologists, restaurant owners, fitness club owners, and supermarket employers. Stakeholders, of course, will vary according to the target problem.

Citizen participation and community partnerships are cornerstones of community health practice. They are not, however, a substitute for systematic assessment and analysis of the community culture matrix. Indeed, the very selection of community members to participate in health planning is a pivotal step that must be grounded in cultural knowledge—not just about who the stakeholders are but to whom they are related, and how. What are their records on committee issues? What are their political affiliations? Are there potential conflicts of interest? Only through an understanding of community culture is it possible to identify and understand the relationships among various individuals and subgroups and how they will play out in community health planning.

CREATING A CULTURE-BASED COMMUNITY HEALTH PLAN

The goal of community health practice is capacity building, i.e., assisting residents to assume ownership of the health and quality of their community. Capacity building requires collaboration among community members to plan for the future. In many localities, both public and private healthcare planning organizations already are in place in the form of health departments, community alliances, strategic planning groups, and associations of care providers. Culture-based planning requires the integration of new initiatives with the existing community planning structure. Thus, it is necessary first to determine the organizations and individuals who currently are responsible for overseeing the health of a community.

As described in Chapter 4, the characteristics of the planning infrastructure and its membership will vary from place to place, reflecting local values and social structures found in the community. Ongoing assessment of the health and culture of the community helps to assure capacity-building plans and activities are coordinated and consistent with the changing needs and characteristics of the community. In addition, there should be protocols for customary articulation with other health- and social-planning groups, both within and outside the community, on the municipal, county, state, and national levels. This helps to assure that local data flow to central planning bodies and are included in shaping public policy so that it is sufficiently flexible to serve local communities.

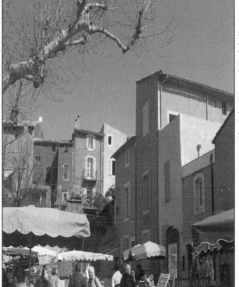

Photo by Bernard Delobelle, France.

Community health nursing is often presented as a linear process in which planning comes after assessment and before implementation. In fact, however, planning is included in every component of community health practice and requires ongoing dialogue with community residents. The kinds of data required for planning must be identified, along with when and how they are to be collected and for what duration. Then projects must be prioritized and scheduled for implementation. In reality, planning is unending, sometimes chaotic, and always responding to new information and change. Therefore, while the following phases of community health planning are presented in a sequential format, all the component activities are likely to occur simultaneously. Planning is a fluid activity in which goals are meant to be revisited routinely throughout the process.

Finally, in addition to knowing the structure, participants, and processes of planning prior to implementation, it is essential to have an understanding of the philosophies and values that guide health planning in a community. An example of a philosophical or value statement is that all people have the right to health. Another philosophical statement is that it is better to prevent disease than to cure it. These are not empirical statements, derived from financial data or observations of the community. Rather, they are reflections of societal and professional values. While such statements acknowledge declared norms, it is in actual practice that the underlying, unspoken values are exposed. Some might say, for example, that a real driving value of contemporary healthcare is that sophisticated and expensive medical procedures will be reserved for those who have the ability to pay.

As presented in Chapter 2, the field of community health has espoused values related to an emphasis on prevention, health promotion, and sustainable communities in which all citizens are engaged. The realities of health disparities (the sanitized word for inequities) and the disenfranchisement of whole sectors of community residents, however, reveal more about our health system than commonly stated values. Moreover, it is possible for people to endorse values in some situations that may be contrary to values they endorse in other situations. Nevertheless, it is useful to acknowledge the range of values—universal and situational—that are linked to health planning.

GOALS

The first step of health planning is the identification of goals. In clinical practice, goals are formulated with an individual or family, based on data derived in the assessment phase. The same is true in community health practice. The community plan is based on the cultural and health assessments outlined in Chapters 3 and 4. Each need or problem must be examined in relation to the cultural context. In *Healthy People 2010,* a number of objectives are identified that, collectively, advance a national agenda for health improvement. It would be misguided, however, to assume any one objective will apply to all communities or that all objectives will apply to any single community. The two major goals of *Healthy People 2010*—to increase the quality and years of healthy life and to eliminate disparities in health (USDHHS, 2001)—are universally applicable, but the implementation will vary with each community.

For example, one of the objectives in *Healthy People 2010* is to eliminate ethnic disparities in high school completion rates. Dropping out of school is associated with deferred employment, poverty, and poor health. By addressing high school dropout rates as part of the nation's health promotion and disease prevention agenda, it may be possible to reduce health risks commonly attributed to specific ethnic groups. The target of 90% set for this objective is consistent with the national education goals to increase the high school graduation rate of all ethnic and racial groups to at least 90%. In 1996, only 62% of Hispanic/Latino and 83% of African-American youth aged 18-24 had completed high school, compared to a completion rate of 92% for white, non-Hispanic youth (USDHHS, 2001).

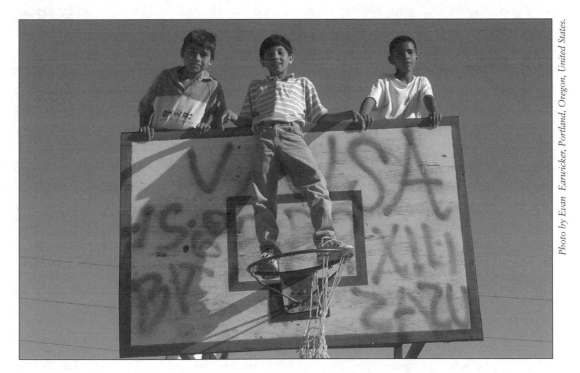

Photo by Evan Earwicker, Portland, Oregon, United States.

While the goal to remove disparities in high school completion rates may apply to many communities, the causes of the problem and the strategies for the solution will be determined by local circumstances. In one community, the disparities in high school completion rates may occur because of the need for young men to assist their families by entering the economy in their teenage years. In another community, the ethnic disparity in high school completion may be linked to a high rate of teenage pregnancy.

To be most effective, goals should be phrased in terms of the desired outcomes rather than the interventions. Framing a goal in terms of the solution reduces the options and limits the community investments. For example, the goal to improve high school completion rates could be framed as "improve the math and writing skills of at-risk adolescents," or "provide sex education for at-risk teenagers." While there is nothing terribly wrong with these goals, they tend to be limited strategically and may engage a fairly narrow segment of the community. In contrast, phrasing it as an outcome, e.g., "the goal is to reduce ethnic disparities in high school completion rates in the community" expands the range of possible solutions and invests more individuals and groups in achieving the goal. Then the goal of increasing high school completion rates in specific groups might engage, for example, school health nurses, educators, politicians, day-care center operators, parents, coaches, employers, college and university officials, religious leaders, and law enforcement personnel.

Goal setting in community health is a determination of the multiple needs and expectations of community members. If local residents remain unconvinced of the importance of a problem, it will be difficult to resolve. Both the goals and the strategies of the plan must be culturally acceptable to those affected. For example, it would be inappropriate in some communities to establish, unilaterally, the strategy of reducing the rate of "adolescent pregnancy" to achieve the goal of 90% high school completion rates. The decision of when to become pregnant is guided by cultural norms related to mating, marriage, and domestic organization. The course of pregnancy also is often guided by religious norms and the socioeconomic situations of the families involved. In communities that are comfortable with teen pregnancy, improving high school completion rates may center on assuring that teen mothers do not encounter barriers to completing high school, rather than on preventing pregnancy.

PRIORITIES

In most circumstances, all the identified needs cannot be met at the same time. But a culturally integrated approach will help create an effective and realistic timeline for fulfilling the community health agenda (Kurtenbach & Warmoth, 1995). This is why it is essential the health plan be grounded firmly in the assessment of community culture, as well as community health. Using the community rather than specific health problems as the focus of planning, the criteria for assigning priority should include (1) the extent of risk to the *entire* community if the problem is unresolved, and (2) the extent to which the solution of one problem will solve many other problems. Ultimately the goal is to build the capacity of communities to address their own health problems, or, better yet, to prevent such problems from occurring. One of the features

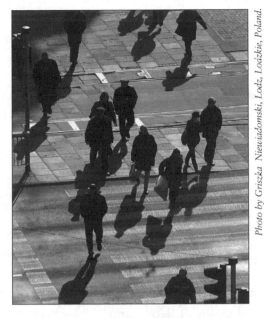

Photo by Griszka Niewiadomski, Lodz, Łoózkie, Poland.

of goal prioritization is forecasting, i.e., determining what would happen if one problem was selected for action as opposed to another. It is also necessary to forecast what would happen if nothing was done about the problem. For example, given the close relationship between education and health, high school completion rates are likely to have a compelling effect on the future health of the community and its population. Although it is impossible to predict the future exactly, the community culture assessment provides a vantage point from which sequences of events can be more accurately forecasted.

In addition to the differences of opinion within the community regarding health and other aspects of social life, there also are differences between providers and lay citizens about health priorities. Residents may feel, for example, that adolescent sexuality is a serious problem, but for the provider community, the rates of STIs and adolescent pregnancy may not be sufficient to warrant programmatic intervention. Epidemiological data, on the other hand, may suggest adolescent smoking is a serious, widespread problem that captures the attention of the providers, but is of less interest to parents and other citizens. The reconciliation of professionally identified needs and community-identified demands is important in developing a culturally integrated strategy for building capacity. Support from community residents is more likely if the plan is sensitive to their expectations and interests. This does not mean goals derived from provider-based assessment of health risks should be forsaken or even placed on hold. It simply means a successful planning strategy should be constructed in a cultural framework that attends to community interests, e.g., a high school education program that addresses sexuality as well as tobacco use and dietary behaviors.

MEASURABLE OUTCOMES

Once the goals have been prioritized, they must be translated into measurable outcomes— specific outcomes that will demonstrate the attainment of a goal. The *Healthy People 2010* objective to eliminate ethnic disparities in high school completion rates is both data-driven (from an analysis of education statistics) and value-driven (from the principles of social equity and justice). The goal must be stated, however, in a way that would make progress measurable. It is better to first ask what specific behaviors or events are desired. The goals would then be phrased in behavioral or measurable terms. *Healthy People 2010* has a target for this objective of at least a 90% high school completion rate for all ethnic groups (USDHHS, 2001).

In addition to stating the target outcomes, it is necessary to state the time frame within which the outcome is expected. The time frame selected will depend on the nature and extent of the problem, the resources available, and the community culture. In some communities, it may be realistic to say ethnic disparities in high school completion rates could

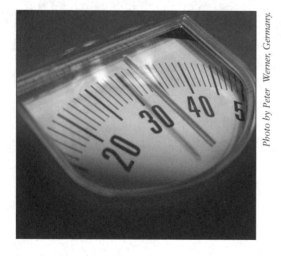

Photo by Peter Werner, Germany.

be eliminated in four years, while others may require a longer period, with interim goals revisited annually. The time frame also should be consistent with the length of time necessary to measure the effects. A reduction in ethnic disparities in high school completion may take much longer than reducing ethnic disparities in obesity. Short-term goals are helpful in providing encouragement to planners and stakeholders when they are successfully accomplished. It is important, however, that long-term, truly consequential goals representing real progress in improving health and reducing disparities not be forgotten in the wake of short-term success.

OPERATIONAL PLANS

An operational plan, or plan of work, designates the specific activities and events that need to occur to achieve the community health goals that were formulated in the previous phase. Goal setting is not limited to the early phases of the community health planning process. As the plan is generated, program goals are translated into a culture-specific plan of work. This is where an understanding of community structure and organization is especially cogent.

Designing a culture-based plan of work, or operational plan, requires exploring the problem against the backdrop of everything that is known about community life: (1) the spatial-temporal dimension, (2) the characteristics of the population, and (3) the social organization. Eliminating the ethnic disparities in high school completion rates, for example, requires exploring the temporal-spatial framework in which teenagers function, i.e., how do they use community space and time?

- Where do they live?

- Where do they get together?

- Where are the high schools located and what are they like?

- How do they organize their time—daily, weekly, seasonally?

- What trends are evident in high school completion?

- Are there ethnic differences in the teenage use of space and time in the community?

Next, the characteristics of the target teens, and how they compare to other populations in the community, is examined.

- Who are the young people who drop out of high school—residence, ethnicity, race, class, religion, gender, age, and so on?

- How are they different from the adolescents who complete high school?

- What reasons do they give for leaving school?

Finally, how the target group fits into the social structure of community life, including class structure and vertical segmentations, is examined, as well as how the target group fits into the various community institutions: religion, education, economic, domestic, recreation.

■ What roles do they occupy in relation to other community institutions—religion, recreation, family, economy, and so on?

■ What are the institutional norms, personnel, and activities that impede, accommodate, or support high school completion for target teens?

■ How do target teens fit into the economic structure of community life?

■ How do target teens fit into the religious institutions?

■ What is the role of target teens within their families?

From this information, a determination is made about how various community institutions, individuals, and groups can be involved in the process of addressing the problem. The activities of the operational plan will be guided by knowledge of the culture. If young people have to leave school to help support their families, the operational plan for that community will be different from one in which a high dropout rate is attributed to other causes. Two communities can manifest the same problems, but the different cultural contexts in which the problem is embedded will mandate different solutions.

Operational plans encompass two kinds of planning. One is called the *activity* plan, which consists of the logical steps one must take to reach a goal or solve a problem. The other is called a *strategic* plan and consists of the activities and events that are needed to manage the context so that the activity plan can be implemented. The activity plan for eliminating ethnic disparities in high school completion might call for helping teenage mothers to continue their education during and after pregnancy. This would permit them to have at least a beginning preparation for earning a livelihood and achieving economic stability for themselves and their children. The strategic plan, on the other hand, might call for enlisting the support of influential community members to convince those parents and teachers who object to the presence of pregnant teenagers in high school.

COST-EFFECTIVENESS

A good community plan offers the most cost-effective solution to the problem (Sullivan, 1990). Cost-effectiveness is not synonymous with least expensive. Rather, it gives consideration to the relationship between cost and quality. For one intervention to be considered more cost-effective than another, it must provide equal outcomes at a lower cost or better outcomes at the same cost. Furthermore, cost must be measured not only in terms of dollars and cents, but in psychological tolls, time, and productivity, which often are difficult to translate into monetary terms. There also are costs incurred by the community if such a program is *not* implemented. Finally, an assessment of costs must be calculated in a time frame and projected over a period of years. While the initial costs may be high, its maintenance may require little investment. On the other hand, a plan with lower start-up costs could ultimately prove to be the more expensive alternative. It is common, for example, to argue that conducting a cultural assessment is too time-consuming and costly. Yet, when the plan is consistent with the cultural expectations and conditions of the community, time-consuming and costly

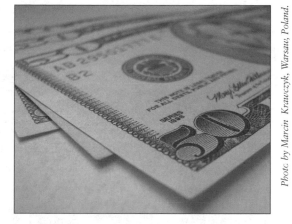

Photo by Marcin Krawczyk, Warsaw, Poland.

problems can be avoided. Identifying and deploying local cultural capital make efficient use of community resources while investing community residents and groups in the plan.

Despite the governmental emphasis on controlling the cost of healthcare through planning, there remain many barriers to comprehensive health planning that increase public expenditures on health. Primary among these is the continuing emphasis on specific health problems rather than on building community capacity, resulting in categorical programs, each with its own funds, facilities, and personnel. This unnecessary fragmentation is both costly and confusing for communities. A related problem in health planning is the lack of integration between health and other community services such as education, recreation, and protective services. Each has its own planning boards, districts, and structures, even though an event in one system is likely to seriously impact the others. A third barrier to health planning is its politicization; the more powerful voices of the community have the opportunity to further entrench health disparities and impede community action.

EVALUATION

Although evaluation is usually thought of as coming at the end of the program, it is important to construct an evaluation protocol during the planning stage that establishes the criteria by which progress will be measured, a timeline for evaluation, and the procedures to be employed (including the who, where, and what). In clinical practice, baseline data on the presence of fever, redness, or swelling tell us whether the treatment has been effective by measuring those criteria at specified periods of time. Community practice has the same requirement for baseline data, for example: In 2001, only 60% of Latino boys completed high school, or in 2001, 37% of adolescents were overweight or obese (USDHHS, 2001).

Unlike clinical practice, however, evaluation in community health is complicated by the length of time usually required to see results of interventions and by the vast number of intervening variables that influence progress.

It is helpful to evaluate progress periodically, rather than waiting until it is completed, so trends and modifications can be determined throughout the designated implementation period. Interim results (often referred to as formative or proxy evaluations) that suggest sufficient progress is not being made provide an opportunity to revisit the operational plan. Finally, the individuals designated as evaluators should not be those who have a vested interest in either the success or failure of the plan. This is not to say those who have a vested interest are incapable of doing an honest evaluation. Rather, it means an evaluation conducted and reported by those who have no stake in a program's success or failure is likely to have more credibility. The final step is to summarize the results and report on the merit of the criteria being evaluated.

CULTURE, CHANGE, AND PLANNING

From the examples in this chapter, it is clear that planning often inspires and is inspired by change. The role of the nurse as a change agent has led some to assume change is inherently good or necessary and should be implemented for its own sake. On the other hand, for many years, community health nurses were guided by the notions that only incremental change is effective change, and rapid change is necessarily injurious to the community. Both notions—that change is inherently good and that rapid change is inherently disorganizing—are problematic, because they have taken change out of context. The nature, extent, and speed of planned change depends on the problems being addressed and the cultural milieu in which they occur. Certainly, rapid change is consistent with the "real time" of contemporary lifestyles; fashions alter drastically from one year to the next, and new technology is being introduced and absorbed at a rate never imagined. Incremental change is often simply a vehicle for maintaining the power structure of the community and protecting vested interests. The mandate is not change, but change for the purpose of ensuring the health of the public through the development of community capacity. This may or may not require major alterations in community life. Before planners determine how change should be accomplished, they must first determine whether change is necessary. The goal of culture-based planning is not to accelerate change nor to restrain it, but rather to manage it with minimal upheaval and cost to the community. A major challenge for contemporary health planners and policymakers is to generate health plans that have sufficient flexibility to survive in a rapidly changing society.

REFERENCES

Bibeau, G. (1997). At work in the field of public health: The abuse of rationality. *Medical Anthropology Quarterly, 11*(2), 246-252.

Clinton, G.A. (1979). *Local success and federal failure: A study of community development and educational change in the rural south.* Cambridge: Abt Books.

Davidge, R.C., & Pearson, V.M. (1995). Healthy vision. *Health Progress, 76*(6), 48-51.

Dreher, M. (1984). District nursing: The cost benefits of a population-based practice. *American Journal of Community Health, 74*(10), 1107-1111.

Ervin, N.E., & Kuehnert, P.L. (1993). Application of a model for community health nursing program planning. *Community Health Nursing, 10*(1), 25-30.

Evans, R.G., & Stoddart, G.L. (1994). Producing health and consuming health care. In R.G. Evans, M.L. Borer, & T.R. Marmot (Eds.), *Why are some people healthy and others not?* New York: Aldine deGruyter.

Ferretti, C.K, Verhey, M.P., & Isham, M.M. (1996). Development of a nurse-managed, school-based health center. *Nurse Educator, 21*(5), 35-42.

Gehlbach, S. (2005). *American plagues: Lessons from our battles with disease.* New York: McGraw Hill.

Gorosh, V. (1995). The role of the international nurse in strategic planning. *Nursing and Health Care: Perspectives on Community, 16*(6), 326-331.

Hill, C. (1988). *Community health systems in the rural American south: Linking people with policy.* Boulder, CO: Westview Press.

Hornberger, C., & Cobb, A. (1998). A rural vision of a healthy community. *Public Health Nursing, 15*(5), 363-369.

Kurtenbach, J., & Warmoth, T. (1995). Strategic planning futurists need to be captivation-specific and epidemiological. *Health Care Strategic Management, 13*(9), 8-11.

Lassiter, P.G. (1992). A community development perspective for rural nursing. *Family and Community Health 14*(4), 29-39.

McClain, J.O. (1978). A model for regional obstetric bed planning. *Health Services Research, (Winter)*, 378-394.

Paine-Andrews, A., Francisco, V.T., & Fawcett, S.B. (1994). Assessing community health concerns and implementing a microgrant program for self-help initiatives. *American Journal of Community health, 84*(2), 316-318.

Quad Council of Public Health Nursing Organizations. (2003). Public health nursing competencies. Retrieved July 1, 2005, from http://astdn.org/publicationquadcouncil-phncompetencies.htm.

Salmon, M.E. (1993). Public health nursing: The opportunity of a lifetime. *American Journal of Public Health 83*(1), 674-675.

Satia, J.K., Mavalankar, D.V., & Sharma, B. (1994). Micro-level planning using rapid assessment for primary health care services. *Health Policy & Planning, 9*(3), 318-330.

Steckler, A.B., & Herzog, W.T. (1979). How to keep your mandated citizen board out of your hair and off your back: A guide for executive directors. *American Journal of Community Health, 69*(8), 809-812.

Sullivan, L.W. (1990). Healthy people 2000: Promoting health and building a culture of character. *American Journal of Health Promotion, 5*(1), 5-6.

U.S. Department of Health, Education, and Welfare. (1974). *Planning & Resources Development Act of 1974 (P.L. 93-641)*. Washington, DC: U.S. Government Printing Office.

U.S. Department of Health and Human Services. (2001). *Healthy people 2010*. McLean, VA: International Medical Publishing, Inc.

Washington, G.T. (1998). *After the flood. Nursing and health care perspectives, 19*(2), 66-71.

White, K.L. (1973). Life and death and medicine. *Scientific American, 229*(3), 23-33.

Yakoob, M., & Whiteford, L. (1994). Behavior in water supply and sanitation. *Human Organization, 53*(4), 330-335.

6

COMMUNITY PRACTICE IMPLEMENTATION: CULTURE-BASED LEADERSHIP

Most of the literature on community health planning and implementation describes the processes involved, but neglects to inform us of the strategies required to manage the almost predictable tensions that occur when working with many people who have various priorities.

Implementation in community health practice is all about leadership. It is taking responsibility for assisting communities to enhance their capacity for a sustainable healthy and robust future. It requires bringing people together for social action and using knowledge about the community culture to advance the health of all citizens. This chapter explores culturally grounded leadership strategies for building community capacity.

CHAPTER 6 OBJECTIVES

- Distinguish between the *conflict* and *consensus* models of public health action.

- Identify the special challenges of working with the community as client and the skills and theories needed.

- Describe the process of building a constituency.

- Describe the process of building a coalition.

- Distinguish between primary and secondary target groups in mobilizing community action.

- Prepare an effective public health message.

IMPLEMENTATION, LEADERSHIP, AND COMMUNITY NURSING PRACTICE

To accomplish the broad, far-reaching changes that will build sustainable healthy communities, community advocacy must include large-scale social action (Atwood, Colditz, & Kaw-achi, 1997; Butterfield, 1990; Cwikel, 1994; Drevdahl, 1995; Milio, 1975). In this chapter, culturally grounded strategies for achieving the goals of *Healthy People 2010* will be explored. The purpose here is not to describe the many kinds of actions that fall under the major approaches, since they are as numerous as the problems that necessitate them. Rather, it is to explore the principles that underlie successful strategies for making those initiatives work.

IMPLEMENTATION STRATEGIES

Most of the literature on community health planning and implementation describes the processes involved, but neglects the strategies required to manage the almost predictable tensions that occur when working with many people who have various priorities. Despite the absence of formulas for action (other than a solid grounding in community culture), there are some basic strategies that have informed public health community partnership efforts. Perhaps best known is the *consensus model* (Rothman, 1979).

The consensus (or integrative) model assumes communities are defined by a common set of core values around which members organize to achieve common goals. Since shared values are the organizing force of this model, it is most effective in communities that are very homogeneous. Consensus goals are centered on achieving community-wide collaboration, including endorsement from the existing power structure. Based on an idealistic view of human relationships and a shared desire for the common good, the methods used in the consensus model are enhancing communication, improving moral and rational persuasion, and building rapport. The perception of communities as groups defined by common values and interests has a long history in public health. It is assumed that members of a community know and interact with each other and share what Rosen (1954) called a minimum

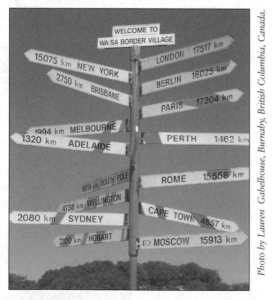

Photo by Lauren Gabelhouse, Burnaby, British Columbia, Canada.

of common interests. This definition has underpinned community health nursing, which by and large has promoted discussion, values clarification, public education, exchange of ideas, and better communication as the vehicles for change. In her conceptualization of the holographic community, Davis (2000) describes communities as "sharing a purpose, acting in unity, and providing nourishment to members" (p. 295).

In contrast, the *conflict model,* or power model (Alinsky, 1971; Jones, 1977), assumes the existence of inherent conflicts in all human groups, including communities. Rather than stressing the commonality among community members, the conflict model emphasizes status differences, competing affiliations, and power relationships. Implementation strategies are generated from the explicit acknowledgement of vested interests, multiple community roles, conflicting values, and power plays. In this model, it is argued that expansive change is likely to require realignment of power rather than consensus (Farley, 1995). Using this model, one seeks to alter the existing decision-making process through social affiliations and political action. The conflict model is based on what some might consider a more cynical view of humanity—that people are guided by self-interest.

These two strategies reflect fundamentally different theories about the nature of communities. One is that communities are held together by an ideology and value system that is shared by its members. The other is that communities are held together by the diversity of values and goals and the capacity of members to meet each other's needs. For example, in a college or university, the students, faculty, and administrators all may have quite different goals, values, and reasons for being there, but they hold the university together through a complex exchange of money, services, and knowledge.

Both models are useful provided they are used appropriately. In spite of substantial and long-standing evidence to the contrary, many continue to assume that all groups can be empowered to take action through community-wide consensus and rational persuasion. Often, however, the change that can be achieved through consensus is relatively trivial and does not address the social and economic dislocations at the root of the problem. The reason people don't want to change is generally not because they have an inherent, psychological resistance to change, but because they have a vested interest in the status quo. Whether change is described as disorganizing or reorganizing depends on where one stands in the shifting control of resources. Thus, while communication and collaboration are essential ingredients of community organization, they may not be sufficient to accomplish the plan in the face of vested interests, power groups, and competition.

The conflict model implies opposition, but it also implies exchange. In the case of a factory, for example, management needs the human labor provided by the workers, and the workers need the income provided by management. In this exchange, both parties give something and get something, but they are motivated by different goals and desires. Change, therefore, can take place by one of the parties withholding what the other wants. On the other hand, the exchange model does not mean doing battle all the time. In fact, it often means building bridges between groups that normally have little contact with one another, so that members can get to know each other as human beings. When this happens, stereotypes are likely to break down and people begin to bring their reference groups together in a spirit of cooperation. These bridges, however, are not generally predicated on like values, good will, and humanitarian interests. Rather, they are predicated on the notion that each group has something the other needs or wants. Thus, by understanding the nature of vested interests, relationships can be facilitated between and among people who can accomplish their own goals while promoting the health of the public. In other words, the way to deal with vested interests is to understand them and use them. Rather than be put off by what may be construed as avarice and opportunism, the presence of self-interest can be acknowledged and used in formulating a strategy that will accomplish the healthy community agenda. It is not uncommon in this model for people to do the right thing for the wrong reason.

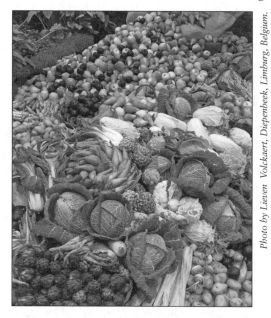

Photo by Lieven Volckaert, Diepenbeek, Limburg, Belgium.

An example of this occurred in an Eastern city where parents requested the city council designate certain blocks as "play" streets, so they could open fire hydrants on hot summer days. Some councilors endorsed this endeavor because they believed that safety and quality of life for children were important. Others had little interest in the project but supported it because their fellow councilors had supported their causes in the past. Thus, a sufficiently broad base of community support countered opposition from residents who felt inconvenienced by the closing of streets.

At first, the conflict model may appear to be Machiavellian or manipulative, but the fact that people differ in their commitment to what has been defined as a worthy cause is simply a reflection of different priorities. Some citizens will support programs for elders but be indifferent to the handicapped; others will support adolescent programs but disregard the homeless. It matters little whether people give money to support a community health project because they believe the project is wholesome or morally right, or because they earn a tax deduction. Similarly, it does not matter much whether a politician supports a public health policy change because it will improve the health of the public, or because it will win votes. The important thing is that community health nurses have been effective in mobilizing the healthy community agenda.

It is also important to remember that what is "right" in community life is seldom black or white. Practically all people live in a world of shifting priorities and contradictions and claim a morality they cannot possibly practice to its fullest. Most people, for example, endorse both freedom of the press and the protection of individual privacy. Yet these two values are often in conflict. If a highly regarded person is the subject of an unflattering front-page story, community residents may find themselves supporting the right to privacy. On the other hand, the same residents may invoke freedom of the press to discredit a less highly regarded individual. According to Bibeau (1997), the lack of success in health promotion and prevention initiatives in North America and throughout the world can be attributed to the failure to acknowledge the complexities of community culture.

No matter which organizational strategy or combination of strategies is used in public health, the goals are achieved by identifying and deploying the cultural capital of the community—values, beliefs, events, organizations, and citizens—to build public health capacity. By articulating community health goals with the community's culture and sharing the responsibility for community health with its residents, the chances for building community capacity are greatly improved. This is true whether the issue is acquiring the resources to prevent domestic violence, cleaning up toxic waste, or establishing a summer recreation program for children.

THE COMPLEXITY OF COMMUNITY CLIENTS

Compared with individual clients, community clients pose special challenges for community health nurses (Omidian & Lipson, 1996). For example, individual patients have relatively predictable organ systems, but the anatomy and physiology of the community client varies stunningly from setting to setting. Community clients are composed of a much less predictable arrangement of people, groups, institutions, classes, and organizations. Also unlike the human organism, which is, relatively speaking, ordered and consistent, these large, unwieldy, complicated, and heterogeneous clients are made up of individuals and groups with manifold and sometimes opposing interests. Indeed, it is seldom the case that an entire community will agree on what needs to be accomplished and in what order.

Community diversity is likely to increase with size, but even the smallest communities may be composed of different factions that impede the ability to achieve a common purpose. More than 50 years ago, for example, Wellin (1955) reported that within a tiny Peruvian village, thought to be homogeneous, there was great variation in the acceptance of innovation (water boiling). In 1978, Pelto and Pelto suggested there frequently is more diversity within a community than there is between or among communities. Yet today, assertions about community homogeneity continue to permeate public health theory and practice (Bibeau, 1997). So-called "rational" public health policies still disregard the inevitable internal differences and inconsistencies in communities, thus jeopardizing public health action. In the *Healthy People 2010* document, for example, "the community" is referred to as if it were composed of individuals who could be identified by common action and shared systems of belief. Ironically, if this were true, there would be no need for the 2010 overarching goal of eliminating health disparities.

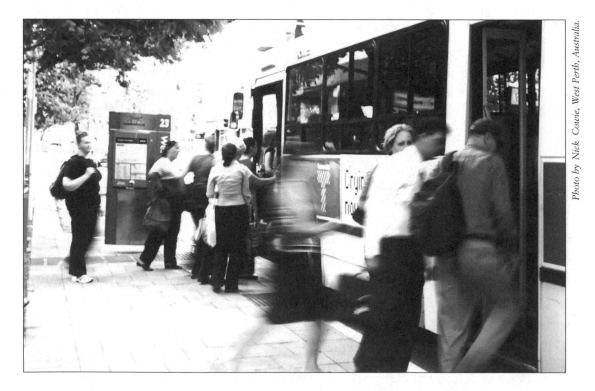

Photo by Nick Cowie, West Perth, Australia.

To be effective in achieving a community health agenda, monolithic descriptions of culture and communities (e.g., "the Navajo community is superstitious and doesn't want outside assistance," or "the inner-city Hispanic community supports the new health center," or "nurses must partner with rural communities") must be contested. Instead, there should be acknowledgement of the diversity in behavior, beliefs, and institutions that is found within all so-called homogeneous communities and groups (Wandersman et al., 1996). It is this internal diversity that makes community assessment imperative.

In addition to their internal diversity, communities vary in their degree of integration. While the citizens of some communities are intensely linked in a network of social and economic relationships, others are more loosely organized. In highly integrated communities, citizens are connected in multiple ways—residence, kinship, job affiliations, church membership, and voluntary associations. Residents enjoy "multiple-interest" relationships in which they not only are neighbors, but also friends, relatives, co-workers, and club members. In contrast, it is common for more transient and larger communities to have a comparatively dispersed organization in which people may live in the same neighborhood, but they work in different locations, their children attend different schools, and their relatives live in distant places. As neighbors, their relationships tend to be more "single-interest." It is possible to scale communities on the degree to which multiple- or single-interest relationships prevail, ranging from small, comparatively homogeneous, long-standing communities in which social relationships are most intense, to larger, more transitory communities in which members are connected in fewer ways.

More integrated communities are not necessarily better or worse than less integrated communities. In fact, the degree of integration may have little impact on whether people get along and like each other. It is simply a consideration in facilitating community action. If the community is highly integrated, as in some small towns and long-standing neighborhoods where families are established over several generations, the ability to effect change will depend greatly on support from traditional community dynasties. If this support can be obtained, the rest of the community is likely to follow. Without such support, however, it may be difficult to solicit widespread endorsement in a community where people are highly connected to one another and have much to lose by taking an opposing position. The same is true of single-industry communities in which the factory or resort or plantation controls the community by virtue of its economic influence. In contrast, less integrated suburban or urban neighborhoods, with their more dispersed power structures, provide more options for action—even though, collectively, they may not be as effective as a single strategy in a more integrated community.

The extent to which success in mobilizing a community for health action is realized depends on knowledge of the community and the ability to reframe implementation according to local culture. Given the cultural dissonance that can occur between nurse and community, this is not always easy. While the same is true in clinical practice, it is comparatively easy to isolate the cultural beliefs and behaviors of patients and their families, work with them, respect them, and then leave them. Public health practice, on the other hand, requires a long-term immersion in communities where the nurse may find it difficult to see the logic of customs, behaviors, and social structures (Eng, Salmon, & Mullan, 1992).

On entering a community for the first time, it is relatively easy to identify its problems and weaknesses and then attribute them to the local culture and social organization. Though it is tempting to want to wipe the slate clean and start all over again, a disregard for the intricate patterns and institutions that have been established over decades—even centuries—would seriously jeopardize the chances for success. Furthermore, many of the features of community life that appear, at first blush, to be problems may, in fact, turn out to be strengths. Indeed, most features of community life are likely to have both a positive and a negative aspect, depending on the perspective of the person affected. Often, behavior that is seemingly irrational becomes perfectly understandable when viewed within the cultural framework of community life.

For example, a community health nurse, concerned with promoting the quality of life for elders in a rural county settlement, volunteered to pick up their medications twice a week at a less expensive national chain pharmacy located in the suburbs of the city where she lived. To the nurse's surprise, however, they all preferred to continue purchasing their medications at a local pharmacy, where they paid significantly more. At first, this behavior appeared to be irrational to the nurse. An assessment of the community's culture, however, revealed the pharmacy was a family-owned business that had served the community for generations. The current pharmacist and her husband lived in the neighborhood and attended the same church as many of their customers. Their children attended the local public school, where the husband taught fifth grade. The pharmacy sponsored many community events and organizations, including a Little League baseball team and a high school girls basketball team. Without the advantages of a volume business, the pharmacy must charge residents more than they would pay through a national pharmacy chain. Yet not to patronize this local business would have offended a well-known family and constituted a serious breach of community culture.

Usually, people internal to the culture understand these subtleties and can cite the value of having a pharmacist who knows you, who is willing to get up in the middle of the night, and who will give you a month to pay, if necessary. Thus, what might be considered irrational health behavior was completely understandable in the context of community culture. The residents of this community had a relationship with their pharmacist. They were committed to her and she to them.

Community health and health-seeking behavior are cultural phenomena and influenced by psychological, social, and economic factors that function independently of health status or health problems. Rather than impugn the existing system or attempt to organize what already is organized, it is important to begin with a more neutral, open position, cultivating relationships within the community and learning the internal logic of community life. There is seldom a need to point out what is wrong with the community to residents who have lived there for generations and are already painfully aware of its failures. Although one may lament the shortcomings of a community culture, to disregard it would be a clear sign of disrespect (Smith-Nonini, 1997). Community health nurses must demonstrate appreciation and respect for the values and traditions of the community client in the same way they would with an individual client—by starting with the community where it is.

Conventional wisdom suggests community advocacy is greatly improved when there is cultural homogeneity between nurse and community, thus minimizing "cultural barriers" to implementation. More recent thinking, however, indicates health providers do not need to be of the same culture as their clients to be effective. Cultural barriers are attributable not so much to the lack of shared experience as they are to poor communication and the absence of a strong personal commitment. Using a community-specific approach, derived from a cultural assessment, the nurse can proceed in a way that is least antagonistic to locally held traditions. This *preservative* approach should not be confused with an incremental or *conservative* approach. The preservative approach is based on the notion that it is possible to accomplish profound and often very rapid change with minimal disruption to local life by casting the change in the context of community culture.

CREATING COMMUNITY RELATIONS: CONSTITUENCIES AND COALITIONS

Being a leader means making things happen. To do this, the community health nurse must have a strong base of support that will sufficiently empower him or her to mobilize communities for social action (Jamieson, 1996; Salber, 1970). Thus, the first step in establishing leadership is to build relationships with local groups and individuals. Generally, these take the form of constituencies and coalitions. Ordinarily, constituencies are thought of in the political sense, as all the people who make up the electorate of a politician. An expanded definition of constituency, however, is a group of people who provide ongoing patronage, support, and representation. In contrast, coalitions are groups of individuals and organizations that convene for the express purpose of accomplishing a specific goal. Both constituencies and coalitions are necessary to facilitate a community health agenda.

Building community relations requires becoming highly visible and known to all segments of the population, meeting and developing relationships with politicians, public officials, religious and education leaders, and influential business people. Drevdahl (1995) has made the point that community health often is entrusted to individuals who have all the right education and credentials, but who lack a relationship with those whom they are supposed to serve. The community health nurse who does not know or is not known by the key members of a community will have a difficult time accomplishing the goals and objectives of the community health plan.

Traditionally, nurses have derived their power from their ministrations. The counsel, care, and comfort they provide to patients and their families both continuously and in times of crisis are a powerful means of establishing and securing relationships. To build a community-wide base of support, however, the nurse's authority must reach beyond the private domain of home and family and into the public arena. Health and illness are matters that have the potential for affecting every member of a community, either directly or indirectly, and community health nurses are experts on how people can stay well and manage health problems. That expertise is an impressive source of influence. As prominent members of the community whose mission is highly valued, nurses easily can acquire grassroots support from families and their community. Most nurses, however, are unaware of the magnitude of the power at their disposal and seldom use it, even though their contact with all sectors of the population provides a range of relationships that would be the envy of any legislator running for office (Jamieson, 1996). Ironically, politicians are acutely aware of the influence nurses command—both as a profession (by the magnitude of its membership) and as individuals who have acquired the admiration, respect, and confidence of community residents.

In clinical practice, nurses understand the significance of establishing relationships with their patients for effective interventions. Eventually, nurses come to know their patients well and to use those relationships therapeutically. But relationship-building with whole communities offers new and interesting prospects, again reflecting the complexity and diversity of community clients. Nurses are accustomed, for example, to establishing a sense of confidence and trust with patients and their families as they become active and essential participants in their plans of care. In community health nursing, it is equally imperative to establish a strong and trusting relationship with clients and engage them in community action. But since communities are composed of competing populations, groups, and institutions, establishing a trusting relationship with one segment of the community could generate distrust in another segment. Therefore, nurses must avoid even the appearance of an exclusive affiliation with one segment that could limit their effectiveness in working with the community as a whole. If, for example, the community health nurse attends a Methodist church, it is particularly important to take the time to meet with the leaders of other religions and denominations, thus demonstrating respect for the beliefs of others.

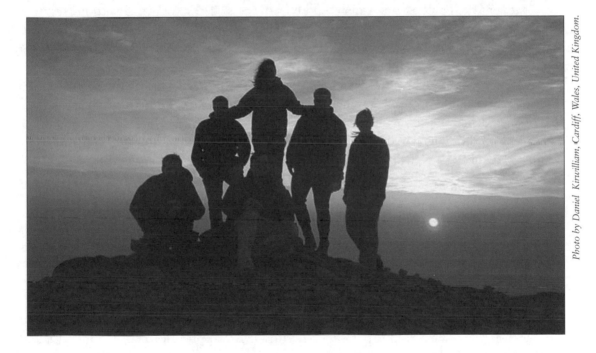

Photo by Daniel Kirwilliam, Cardiff, Wales, United Kingdom.

Community practitioners become, in effect, ex officio members of the community. Nurses are not, however, just any community member. Nurses occupy a special role, relative to other residents, that carries both privileges and obligations. On the one hand, they have more personal freedom than other comparable members of the community and typically are judged by a different set of standards. For example, nurses are permitted—even expected—to develop relationships with all members of the community, including its out-casts, and to visit areas of the community that would be considered off-limits to some residents. They also are privileged to ask highly personal questions and to explore the more intimate details of people's lives. On the other hand, the nurse's position and special role within the community carry certain constraints and responsibilities. Because nurses are reservoirs of knowledge about the personal aspects of residents, they are not privileged to participate in the casual gossip and speculation afforded to most members of the community, without seriously undermining their credibility and the community's confidence.

Building community relations becomes more complicated when community health nurses reside in the community where they work. As residents, nurses are more complex stakeholders, ordinarily occupying several positions or roles that could result in conflicting allegiances. At the same time, participation in community life, especially if a resident, can augment the nurse's commitment and effectiveness. If community health nurses have children attending local schools, for example, they will have a personal, as well as professional, interest in street safety and school health. If related to the owner of the local industry, the nurse may be in a useful position to promote the health of employees. For such community health nurses, the residents of the community are not just their target population; they are their children's teachers, their spouse's employer, their rabbi, or their mechanic. For the residents, the community health nurse is not just a nurse, but also a neighbor, customer, or club member. It is not impossible for resident nurses to build constituencies; it simply requires consideration of these advantages and disadvantages.

Depending on community size, diversity, and complexity, community health nurses may occupy the same position but act out their roles quite differently. Like physicians, social workers, or other human service providers, nurses are guided by an ethos to treat all clients in a consistent manner, regardless of status or background. They should refuse to take into account that clients may be their friends, that their parents are from the same town, or that they live in the same apartment complex. This *universalistic* approach to clients is more likely to be found in the larger, less integrated communities where single dimension relationships prevail. If, on the other hand, the client is a cousin or a neighbor and gets special attention, this is called a *particularistic* approach to clients. It could be especially poor attention or especially good attention, but it is, in any case, special. Particularistic treatment is more common in small, long-standing, integrated communities where multiple-dimension relationships prevail.

Each kind of community poses a different challenge for building community alliances. In one case, the challenge is to develop a structure that will engage members of the community where multiplex relationships and cross-cutting social ties ordinarily do not prevail. In the other, it is to break through the potential patronage that exists in small communities and establish an ambiance of equal participation. While particularistic relationships that exist between nurses and citizens can be beneficial, they also can be offset by the possibility of prejudicial treatment. At the same time, the fairness and professionalism of universalistic relationships in less integrated communities frequently are compromised by depersonalization and indifference.

Achieving effective community rapport means identifying and acknowledging the existing power structure. This includes both the power derived from community position and control of resources, as well as the influence of power often found in informal leadership. An example of the former is a local industrialist who may or may not be well-liked, but who, in fact, controls the economic opportunities available to community residents. Politicians and religious functionaries who have acquired influence through their positions are similar examples, although they may have acceded to that position as a result of popular leadership. In contrast, leadership can be generated from the ranks and based on the charismatic qualities of a particular individual, rather than on his or her formal position within the community. Practically every neighborhood, community, or workplace has a few individuals who are especially well-regarded and influential, even though they control few resources. Because such leaders frequently do not occupy formal positions within the community power structure, they may be more difficult to identify but are no less significant.

Neither source of power can be disregarded in building constituencies or coalitions. There is, however, a tendency on the part of some human service providers to unquestioningly identify with those considered to be disenfranchised and powerless and to exclude the powerful, who are alleged to be the genesis of all the social dislocations and injustices in the community. While, no doubt, there are many cases in which this observation is entirely appropriate, such conclusions should be based on a thorough cultural assessment and analysis. Moreover, oversimplified politics can lead to oversimplified—even naïve—strategies. The net effect of ignoring or antagonizing the power elite of a community may be to alienate those very members of the community who have both the resources and the will to improve the health of the public. The history of community health nursing is full of examples, including the work of Florence Nightingale and Lillian Wald, where great change was accomplished because of influence and philanthropic support from the upper classes (Monteiro, 1985; Spradley & Allender, 1996). The inclusion of the community's elite among the nurse's supporters does not preclude the ability to take social action and realign the existing power structure.

One of the most important vehicles used by community practice nurses to engage the influential members of a community is a community advisory board. The choice of whom to invite to serve on an advisory board should derive directly from the roles and positions of these individuals in relation to the community culture and the means at their disposal for assisting the nurse in building a power base (Rebello, 1995). The real value of such boards is not widespread citizen participation, nor even representation. Those goals can be achieved in a number of other ways. Rather, the boards should serve as brokers or facilitators to help nurses expand their influence. As mentioned in Chapter 5, members typically are drawn from the local power structure and are likely to sit on other community boards as well. This cadre of professional board members, who are sufficiently powerful to control the distribution of resources for health and social services, can be extremely helpful in connecting community nurses to the powerful decision-makers of the community.

Like the human organism, in which organ systems are linked with behavioral dimensions, communities also are matrices in which various institutions and populations intersect. Thus, building community relationships requires attention not only to health institutions, but also to all sectors of community life that will support community capacity building. Assisting local women to become community stakeholders who will build community capacity, for example, requires attending not only to their health, but helping to improve their high school completion rates, providing meaningful employment opportunities, and assisting them to acquire affordable housing. To make this happen, nurses must extend their presence into the educational, commercial, and housing institutions of the community. To build truly powerful constituencies and coalitions, community health nurses must sit on advisory boards in the diverse sectors of the community—for example, the city finance committee, the community planning committee, or the board of education. The various roles and multiple positions charismatic leaders, politicians, religious leaders, health professionals, and board members hold in the community—and how they are linked to one another—are key factors as nurses go about establishing community relations.

IMPLEMENTING THE HEALTHY COMMUNITY AGENDA

A healthy community agenda, like the *Healthy People* agenda, will consist of overarching goals and a number of objectives to be accomplished within given time frames. Implementation embraces both the activity plans and the strategic plans described in Chapter 5. The goal of the activity plan may be to establish a comprehensive health/work/study program for teenagers. In contrast, the strategic plan may be concerned with ways to solicit and expand community support for the project and overcome opposition. Each plan gives rise to two kinds of target populations, or stakeholders, needed to engage a community health plan. The activity plan is directed at the primary target, the category of individuals for whom the program is intended—senior citizens, for example, or migrant workers, or the residents of a specific neighborhood. The secondary target consists of those people and organizations that may not benefit from the program directly, but are somehow instrumental in facilitating

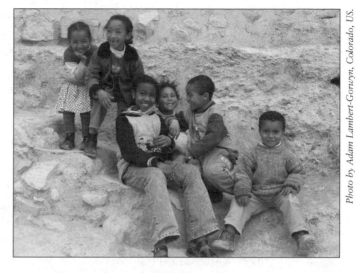

Photo by Adam Lambert-Gorwyn, Colorado, US.

it. Politicians, for example, constitute an important secondary target group in promoting legislation that will provide better housing to the elder residents of a community. Likewise, factory owners may be a critical secondary target group in promoting child health programs for their employees, and children may be the secondary targets for persuading parents to endorse a smoke-free environment policy. Both primary and secondary stakeholders are important for removing barriers to change and mobilizing people to take action.

Secondary targets often include community decision-makers and influential people who are needed to accomplish the proposed plan, as well as those who have a vested interest in the project (Macdonald & Glantz, 1997; Singleton & Hurst, 1996). For instance, if a nurse was planning a state-funded, school-based comprehensive health program for adolescents (the primary target), he or she would want to include representatives from the board of education, the school principal, the president of the high school parent-teacher association, and funding agency representatives, all of who are needed to make the initiative successful. And finally, there are others who may not be essential for implementing the plan, but who have a vested interest in adolescent health and behavior. These might include high school coaches, teachers, the police, mall merchants, school nurses, religious leaders, politicians, members of the recreation departments of city government, and employers of teens, such as restaurant and grocery store owners. These individuals and organizations may have different reasons for being part of the coalition, but their efforts dramatically improve the project's chances for success.

Selecting a coalition is an important part of community health problem-solving, and the effectiveness of a coalition is directly related to the thoroughness of the community assessment. To determine the points at which the target population intersects with the larger community, it is useful to chart the features of the primary target according to the three components of community cultural assessment: (1) time and space, (2) population, and (3) social organization. A project focused on adolescent health, for example, requires the number and proportion of adolescents in the community be known, how they use time and space in the community, the community norms that govern their behavior, and how they fit into the local social structure, including their community roles and responsibilities. In some neighborhoods and small towns, teenagers may be at the center of community life. High school sporting events, homecoming weekends, and proms are organizing events of community cultural life and are deeply embedded in the annual cycle of community activities. In addition to being a focal point of community social life, teenagers may have economic value as wait staff in restaurants, as baby sitters, summer workers, or checkout clerks in grocery stores. In such a community, universal interest in this age group is evident. In other places, however, adolescents are simply another subpopulation that draws little or no attention, as in a large city, where high schools may not be an organizing force in the community.

Thus, while the activity plans (driver education, high school completion, sexual health promotion, and nutritional instruction) may be the same from community to community, the strategic plan and secondary targets will vary according to the role of the primary target in relation to the larger community. Strategic plans should derive directly from knowledge of the community culture: its dimensions of time and space, population characteristics, and social structure. Time, for example, is a critical consideration in forming a coalition. The choice of which politicians to engage in a particular public health project will depend not only on their voting histories and campaign promises, but on the proximity of the next election. The role of the primary target group in the community does not make it necessarily more or less difficult to accomplish the goals. It simply makes the strategies different. For example, in communities where teenagers are not the focus of social activity, it will be difficult to convince community residents to support the plan. Yet a coalition of influential community members may be amazingly successful in persuading other residents to join them in accomplishing their goal. On the other hand, in communities where teenagers are central to local life, there may be so many personal agendas and opinions that getting community members simply to agree on the proposed goals, much less to accomplish them, may be very difficult.

A comparison of two communities, fictionally called "Northville" and "Southfield," located in the same rural county, reveals the way in which the position and role of the target groups influence the strategy for implementation and shape the formation of a coalition.

Nurses from the county decided to seek fiscal support from its 20 towns to extend preventive and health maintenance services to the growing population of elders. Each of the towns already provided a range of well-child services, administered by public health nurses. The services included selected post-natal visits, parenting classes, child development programs, and nutrition programs, as well as immunizations, physical exams, and auditory and vision screenings. These programs were supported with funds derived partly from the state and partly from the collection of town tax revenues. The proposed plan would have expanded public health services to elders and added health education, recreational programs, and community safety to the annual flu prevention programs.

Southfield was a rural farming community with a population of about 2,100 people, of which almost 300 were over the age of 65. Northville, a neighboring community, had a population of about 2,600, of which approximately 250 were over the age of 65. In spite of the demographic similarities between the towns and their geographic proximity, the proposal for a commitment to elder services was accepted readily by elected officials in Southfield but rejected in Northville.

An examination of the role and status of the elder population (the primary target) in each community provided some clues to explain the difference in commitment to the program by each community. Southfield was a farming community in which elders continued to work in some capacity on family-operated farms, assuming, for example, household and child-care responsibilities. Although they may have been less active than their children and/or grandchildren in farm operations, they typically were owners of the farms that succeeding generations would inherit. For the most part, the social life of Southfield was intergenerational and organized around

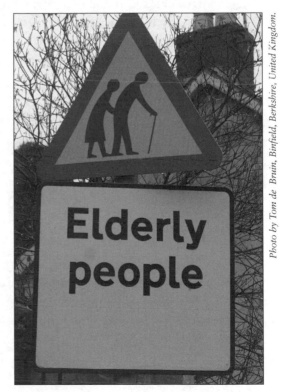

Photo by Tom de Bruin, Binfield, Berkshire, United Kingdom.

the network of extended families that comprised the population of the town. In addition to their central economic roles as owners of the farms, elders continued to take an active role as leaders in town government, church functions, and community social activities, such as the annual fair or the breakfast sponsored by the volunteer firefighters.

Northville resembled Southfield in physical appearance and would have been classified as rural by most standards. Only a small segment of the Northville population still engaged in farming, however, and most of the land was rented to farmers in surrounding communities. Much of the population was employed at the large, prestigious Valley Preparatory School tucked into the hills surrounding the center of town. Since residence in Northville entitled local children to tuition benefits as day students at Valley School, many young families had moved to Northville but commuted daily to work in the county seat located 15 miles away. A few of the elders in this community were senior members of farm families, as in Southfield, but most were retired members of the faculty and staff from the preparatory school. Unlike the elders in Southfield, most in Northville lived far from their sons and daughters who were typically professionals living in other parts of the country. The social and recreational activity of Northville was much more age-segregated, in which the various generations mixed only infrequently. Although both the retired and the younger men engaged in golf as a pastime, the seniors used a local nine-hole course, while the younger men traveled to a more sophisticated golf club in the county seat that put them in contact with their daily business associates.

In comparison with Southfield elders, those in Northville were not well-integrated with the other generations. They played almost no role in town government, which generally was controlled by the younger generation, and had little economic authority in the community. Seniors simply were not a high priority in Northville, and there was even occasional resentment expressed regarding senior residents who continued to occupy large homes in a community where spacious houses were much in demand by young families with children. Essentially, Northville elders had comparatively little authority and few advocates.

This example demonstrates it is not just the size and nature of the target group, but its role and status in relation to the rest of the community—particularly the power structure. In Southfield, where elders were comparatively powerful, town officials readily accepted and implemented the proposal. In Northville, on the other hand, where there was no clearly visible base of support for the retired members of the community, the first step was to identify those groups and individuals who would constitute a coalition.

An analysis of the position of elder community members in relation to the cultural context of Northville revealed various points at which elders did, in fact, intersect with other age groups. First, while they were not great in number, there were a few extended farm families in which grandparents and great-grandparents played a significant role. Second, the Congregational Church, in which some retired faculty members from Valley School served as Sunday school teachers, was one of the few community domains in which intergenerational activities and relationships had developed and flourished—particularly among the women. Third, as leader of a major "industry" in Northville, the headmaster of Valley School was considered to be one of the more influential members of the community.

From this analysis, a Northville coalition was formed that included the following people: (1) the minister of the Congregational Church; (2) a well-liked mother (whose child attended Sunday school at the church and whose husband happened to be an elected town official); (3) a respected farmer whose extended family, including his father, lived on the family farm; and (4) an articulate retired Valley School faculty member. Together, they visited the headmaster of Valley School to ask for his support in convincing town counsel members to provide revenue for the project. His own political leverage stemmed from the school's role as a major employer in the community and from its generous tuition benefits to town children. In the meantime, the wife of the town official convinced her husband to reverse his original opinion on the project, and the much beloved and highly influential minister asked his parishioners for their endorsement. By developing a strategy grounded in knowledge about community culture, this strategically selected coalition was able to overcome the original opposition and secure the resources needed to acquire the commitment of town revenues for promoting the health of seniors.

Typically, a healthy community agenda will be variably received, with some community residents endorsing the entire agenda and others endorsing only parts of it. Each component of the plan is likely to generate enthusiasm in some cases, indifference in others, and opposition in still others. Organizing those who support the initiative is only part of the coalition-building process. It is also necessary to address those who are likely to oppose the initiative and those who are neutral. Neglecting to do so jeopardizes the proposed program, particularly if the opposition is organizing for counteraction. To predict the strategies opponents may employ, identification is made not only of who will resist the plan but also their reasons for resisting it and the extent and nature of influence they have in the community. Using cultural information, community practice nurses develop strategies to persuade, counter, or compromise.

Sometimes opposition is the product of a simple lack of understanding of the project's mission that can easily be corrected with new information and education. In other situations, the reasons are more deep-seated and potentially threatening. For example, a program focusing on adolescent health may be seen as a worthy project, but one that competes with other worthy programs for limited funds. In such a case, it is difficult to generate enthusiasm from those working in other human services and healthcare agencies that ordinarily would be allies. Owners of fast-food and pizza restaurants may anticipate a decline in business and raise objections to the program. Some parents may endorse a program in general, but oppose the specific components that deal with contraception. Both the support and the opposition to capacity-building initiatives are embedded in the social and economic structures that make up the local culture. By identifying the cultural meaning of the objections, it often is possible to construct a trade-off or compromise, or even a "win-win" that will satisfy the opposition and cause them to withdraw their objections.

In any case, it is important not to be lulled into a false sense of security by the inherent logic of the proposal. Even though a program makes sense, it is necessary to be aware that some sectors of the community derive benefits from the system as it currently functions and therefore will oppose the change. It is unlikely a particular behavior or institution would continue to flourish if someone did not stand to gain from it. Therefore, it is best to anticipate there will be opposition to even the most modest and seemingly rational change, and to prepare for it accordingly. Ironically, deterrents to change often may come from health professional groups that have a vested interest in keeping health status and services as they currently exist. Some school nurses, for example, have observed that pediatricians have been forceful opponents of school-based health programs.

The neutral category of community members is equally significant in organizing for action. These are the groups and individuals who have—or believe they have—nothing to gain or lose by the proposed plan and are, therefore, indifferent. This category of community members is particularly important, because it may not be possible to persuade the opponents of a plan to shift their position. Therefore, the support derived from the neutral group may be critical for the project's approval. Furthermore, since these individuals and organizations are irresolute, they could just as easily be persuaded to join the opposition. By including neutral but powerful individuals and organizations in the coalition, neutrality or even apathy may be transformed into commitment. In some cases, a way may be discovered in which the neutral person will stand to benefit directly from the proposed project. In other cases, the benefits will be indirect—such as the repayment of a favor or the opportunity to participate with a coalition of influential members of the community. Thus, the reward may be different for each person or group, but it should represent some form of gain.

The effectiveness with which community health nurses identify and use cultural capital is grounded in their knowledge of the community culture and in their relationships with community members. This does not need to be a complex undertaking. For example, a community health nurse in a northern tourist community asked a local ski resort to donate used ski poles to assist elder residents to walk on the icy streets in winter. In another case, the community health nurse established a free source of home health equipment for residents by asking families to donate hospital beds, commodes, and other equipment acquired during the illness of a family member. He then recruited retired community residents to service and repair them. Ultimately, they were distributed to uninsured individuals and families who could not afford to purchase or rent the equipment.

In any ongoing negotiation, allies, opponents, and neutrals do not remain the same but shift in relation to the problem at hand. Just because the religious leadership supported the establishment of an after-school adolescent recreation program does not mean it will endorse plans for a school-based contraception program. Thus, the allies of one project may be neutral about another and oppose yet another. While at first this shifting posture in relation to the healthy community agenda may seem unwieldy, eventually the nurse has the opportunity to work on behalf of every sector of the community and encourage the participation of all citizens. The nurse can, for example, solicit support from a group that is neutral on one issue by promising support on another to which it is more committed. Similarly, the nurse may have to compromise on a particular effort but will use that compromise in the future by trading it for support to accomplish another community health goal.

Community health nurses articulate and balance competing segments of the community to accomplish healthy community agendas. This activity is what Bailey (1958) called "small politics," or the decisions one makes about relationships and the use of local resources. Small politics does not refer to partisan politics (although community health nurses must be knowledgeable about and involved in partisan politics). Rather, it refers to negotiating effectively within the complex cultural matrix of community life, attending to all segments, and perhaps even exploiting (instead of ignoring) the rivalry among them to move the capacity-building agenda forward. This "score card" of "trade-offs" in community health is the stuff of small politics. Each coalition is composed of a different set of individuals who may have been opponents in the past, but who have come together for a cause they now have in common and who, in the future, may once again find themselves on opposing sides. When various parties have the opportunity to collaborate on some issues, they develop personal relationships that may soften their disagreement on others. Coalitions are important vehicles not only for accomplishing a particular plan, but also for establishing relationships where none existed previously and for engaging all citizens as stakeholders in building community constituencies, coalitions, and capacity. Coalitions are cultural capital.

THE CASE STATEMENT: FORMULATING THE CULTURALLY EFFECTIVE MESSAGE

In clinical practice, nurses communicate treatment plans to their patients in a manner that will convince them that following the plan is in their best interest. This requires individualizing the plan so it is consistent with the lifestyle and values of the specific patient. Similarly, in preparing a case statement, community practice nurses must construct a message that is framed within the cultural experience of the community, thus converting a professionally identified problem or need to a culturally defined demand or issue to create awareness in the community and generate public action. Whether trying to improve working conditions of migrants, control solid waste, or limit smoking in public places, without this consciousness-raising, the community may have little interest in the program, either as recipient or as a facilitator. A contemporary health problem, for example, that has received signifi-

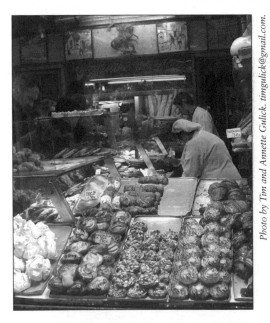

Photo by Tim and Annette Gulick. timgulick@gmail.com.

cant media attention is violence against women. Yet, in the not-so-distant past, violence against women was often unquestioned and even legal in some places. Nurses working in this field have played a major public health role in turning a professionally identified health problem, domestic violence, into a social issue (Dienemann, Campbell, Landenburger, & Curry, 2002). The message in the case statement, as framed, must transform problems into social issues around which coalitions can be mobilized to take action.

It should not be surprising that the community's health alone may not be a sufficiently powerful motivator for public action. The argument that environmental pollution is gradually reducing the ozone layer simply is not as compelling to the average individual as the prospect of losing a job within the next six months because of new regulations governing the disposal of industrial wastes (Hopkins & Mehanna, 2000). Thus, the case statement must identify what will be a more significant justification for supporting a particular health agenda. One innovative community health nurse, for example, "sold" a workers health education and promotion plan to several local industries on the basis of its capacity to reduce absenteeism and disability claims and increase productivity. If the nurse had relied solely on a health promotion message to convince management, it might have failed. Rather than being disappointed by the company's greater interest in worker performance than worker health, the nurse articulated the relationship between them to acquire the support of management.

Given the diversity of the community and the presence of proponents, opponents, and neutrals surrounding almost all capacity-building agendas, the case statement may have to contain more than one message. Some sectors of the community, for example, will respond very well to the argument that regulating the disposal of industrial wastes will result in a healthier environment for future generations. Others will see such an effort as endangering their economic livelihood by regulating the industries in which they work. Still others will be indifferent. In a diverse community, the message must be "segmented" to address the various goals and values of those the nurse is attempting to persuade.

In addition to a culturally appropriate message, the case statement must include the basic facts surrounding the issue. Obviously, politicians cannot disclose they are voting for a piece of legislation because it will win votes in upcoming elections. They must have at their disposal compelling justification for this piece of legislation and how it will benefit their constituents. Thus, case statements consist of (1) a statement of the problem; (2) the number and characteristics of the individuals and families directly affected; (3) the way in which the community is affected, including the cost; (4) the source of the problem; and (5) its proposed resolution. The document should be generated by the coalition and then used to inform all relevant community members, so everyone involved will be working toward the same goal with the same information. While the goal of the case statement is to convince and persuade, all information must be accurate, reliable, and understandable to all. Statistics and statements of fact must be current and compiled from credible sources, checked, and rechecked. Even the most minor math error detracts from the credibility of the document and its authors. Since skeptics will check for any discrepancies in an attempt to discredit the message, the nurse must be prepared to defend the statement and counter arguments.

Finding a proper balance of statistical data and qualitative descriptions will depend on the characteristics of the audience. Since this is a society enamored with numbers, it is useful to include at least a few statistics, but they should be well-chosen and dramatic.

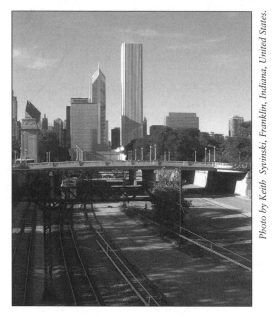

Photo by Keith Syvinski, Franklin, Indiana, United States.

Equally convincing, however, are human-interest data that have an emotional appeal. A description of one or two actual cases often will be more persuasive than the statistics derived from a study of hundreds of families. Thus, while it is necessary to have on hand an objective, rational argument about why a specific plan would improve the health of the community, an emotional appeal is extraordinarily effective, even with the most conservative audience. For example, although figures stating the millions of tax dollars spent on drug abuse each year constitute important evidence, they are somehow less real than the case of a family that lost its home and savings because of drug abuse by one of its members. The plight of real people is something with which most everyone can identify.

SUMMARY

This chapter has contained a description of how community practice nurses assist communities to organize for public health, using leadership skills grounded in an understanding of the local culture. Often, community nursing practice is described as facilitating health through "partnerships" with the community (Mooney & Rambur, 1996). While community partnerships have become the signature of community health practice, they have been regarded with increasing skepticism (Drevdahl, 1995). First, partnerships are exceedingly difficult to operationalize when dealing with entities such as communities, which are amorphous and constantly shifting. Partnerships with individuals and even with formal organizations are feasible because someone is accountable for meeting the terms of the agreement, but how does one "partner" with a whole community? If not the whole community, then with whom—e.g., local government, nongovernmental organizations, block associations? Second, what are the characteristics of such partnerships? How are they constructed and who is responsible for what? Does the preoccupation with being an "equal" partner potentially diminish the expert contribution of the community health nurse? In an even more cynical view, Smith-Nonini (1997) questions whether so-called "partnership coalitions" truly are dedicated to building community capacity or simply are vehicles for persuading citizens to adopt practices advocated by health professionals.

The role of the nurse in building community capacity is not just establishing partnerships with communities to solve identified health problems. Rather, it is a perpetual activity that begins with assembling and maintaining an inventory of the community's cultural capital and continues with engaging individuals and organizations in building community capacity. Just as clinical nurses are responsible for collecting and deploying comprehensive knowledge about patients and families, community health nurses are the custodians of knowledge about the community. Nurses are the members of the health team accountable for gathering, organizing, and updating cultural information and then using it to enhance the public's health. Creating a sustainable healthy community equipped to accommodate opportunities and manage problems as they occur requires not only a plan, but also a sufficient state of readiness and flexibility that is grounded in culturally informed leadership.

REFERENCES

Alinsky, S. (1971). *Rules for radicals*. New York: Vintage Books, Random House.

Atwood, K., Colditz, G.A., & Kawachi, I. (1997). From public health science to prevention policy. Placing science in its social and political contexts. *American Journal of Public Health, 87*(10), 1603-1606.

Bailey, F.G. (1958). *Caste and economic frontier: A village in Highland Orissa*. Highlands, NJ: The Humanities Press.

Bibeau, G. (1997). At work in the fields of public health: The abuse of rationality. *Medical Anthropology Quarterly, 11*(2), 246-255.

Butterfield, P.G. (1990). Thinking upstream: Nurturing a conceptual understanding of the societal context of health behavior. *Advances in Nursing Science, 12*(2), 1-8.

Cwikel, J.G. (1994). After epidemiological research: What next? Community action for health promotion. *Public Health Reviews, 22*, 375-394.

Davis, R. (2000). Holographic community: Reconceptualizing the meaning of community in an era of health care reform. *Nursing Outlook, 48*(6), 295-301.

Dienemann, J., Campbell, J., Landenburger, K., & Curry, M.A. (2002). The domestic violence survivor assessment: A tool for counseling women in intimate partner violence relationships. *Patient Education and Counseling, 46*(3), 221-228.

Drevdahl, D. (1995). Coming to voice: The power of emancipatory community interventions. *Advances in Nursing Science, 18*(2) 13-24.

Eng, E, Salmon, M.E., & Mullan, F. (1992). Community empowerment: The critical base for primary health care. *Family and Community Health, 15*(1), 1-12.

Farley, S.S. (1995). Leadership for developing citizen professional partnerships. *Nursing and Health Care: Perspectives on Community, 16*(4), 226-228.

Hopkins, N., & Mehanna, S.R. (2000). Social action against everyday pollution in Egypt. *Human Organization, 59*(2), 245-254.

Jamieson, M. (1996). Grass roots efforts: Nurses involved in the political process. In E. Cohen (Ed.), *Nurse case management in the 21st century* (pp. 21-27). St. Louis: Mosby.

Jones, D.M. (1977). Strategy straddling: A community organization dilemma in an Alaskan native village. *Human Organization, 36*(1), 22-32.

Macdonald, H., & Glantz, S.A. (1997). The defeat of Philip Morris' "California Uniform tobacco control act." *American Journal of Public Health, 87*(12), 1989-1996.

Milio, N. (1975). *The care of health in communities*. New York: Macmillan.

Monteiro, L. (1985). Florence Nightingale on community health nursing. *American Journal of Public Health, 75*(2), 181-186.

Mooney, M.M., & Rambur, B. (1996). Finding our place at the table. *Nursing and Health Care Perspectives on the Community, 17*(5), 251-254.

Omidian, P.A., & Lipson, J.G. (1996). Ethnic coalitions and public health: Delights and dilemmas with the Afghan health education project in northern California. *Human Organization, 55*(3), 355-360.

Pelto, P.J., & Pelto, G.H. (1978). Anthropological Research. The Structure of Inquiry. New York: Cambridge University Press.

Rebello, A. (1995). Voluntary boards must play leadership role in health reform. *Leadership in Health Services, 4*(2), 8-9.

Rosen, G. (1954). The community and the health officer—A working team. *American Journal of Public Health, 44*(1), 14-16.

Rothman, J. (1979). Three models of community organization practice, their mixing and phasing. In F.M. Cox, J.L. Erlich, J. Rothman, & J.E. Tropman (Eds.), *Strategies of community organization* (pp. 25-45). Ithaca, IL: F.E. Peacock Publishers.

Salber, E.J. (1970). Community participation in neighborhood health centers. *New England Journal of Medicine, 283*(10), 515-520.

Singleton, E.K., & Hurst, C. (1996). Coalition building: A strategy for creating HIV/AIDS awareness on a college campus. *ABNF Journal, 7*(2), 42-46.

Smith-Nonini, S. (1997). Primary health care and its unfulfilled promise of community participation: Lessons from a Salvadoran war zone. *Human Organization, 56*(3), 364-373.

Spradley, B., & Allender, J.A. (1996). *Community health nursing. Concepts and practice* (4th ed.). Philadelphia: Lippincott.

Wandersman, A., Valois, R., Ochs, L., de la Cruz, D.S., Adkins, E., & Goodman, R.M. (1996). Toward a social ecology of community coalitions. *American Journal of Health Promotion, 10*(4), 299-307.

Wellin, E. (1955). Water boiling in a Peruvian town. In B. Paul (Ed.), *Health, culture and community* (pp. 71-103). New York: Russell Sage Foundation.

EPILOGUE

In 1999, the Institute of Medicine published *To Err Is Human: Building a Safer Health System,* the first in a series of reports on the breaches of quality in contemporary American healthcare. It was soon followed by *Crossing the Quality Chasm* (2001) and subsequent volumes that called for an improved healthcare system, girded by changes in the education of health professionals (Institute of Medicine, 2003a) and reorganization of nursing services (Institute of Medicine, 2003b). It should be apparent by now, however, that the health of populations in communities cannot be fixed simply by improving an ailing healthcare system. The goals of *Healthy People 2010,* to extend the quality and years of healthy life and eliminate health disparities, are not just healthcare goals; they are moral imperatives, guided by the ideals of social justice and realized through social activism.

Before the authors of this book fully understood there is no direct relationship between the quality of personal health services and the health of a community, we took great solace in caring for individuals and families in hospitals, homes, schools, industry, and long-term care facilities. Indeed, the heady experience of doing something that was immediately meaningful—even critical—was the allure of nursing right from the get-go. But gradually and inevitably, each of us suffered the frustration of treating clients with illnesses that need not have occurred, or resolving family and developmental problems that were the direct and indisputable outcomes of social and economic dislocations and inequalities.

We were betrayed, in fact, by our own paradigm. The arsenal of concepts and theories that guided our practices was focused almost exclusively on the care of individuals. Derived predominantly from anatomy, physiology, and psychology, the nursing model simply was not sufficient for the far-reaching social change necessary to promote the health of the public and bring an end to health disparities. At the same time, the bodies of knowledge useful for transforming unhealthy places into healthy ones, such as political science, anthropology, sociology, and economics, were typically regarded as incidental to "real" nursing, which took place in intensive care units. The conflicting ideologies generated by these divergent sources of knowledge have been chronicled frequently in the annals of public health nursing, and observers (Freeman, 1963; Williams, 1977; Dreher, 1982; Butterfield, 1990; Drevdahl, 1995) have over the decades acknowledged—and lamented—the disconnect between the *goals* of community nursing (a healthy public in healthy communities) and the *strategies* (personal health services).

While the inherent tension in community practice remains as nurses struggle to meet the needs of both individuals and the public, the *polarizing* effect of these seemingly opposing orientations need not be *paralyzing*. As health activists, community health nurses stand uniquely and pivotally at the intersection of biological and social sciences, where the good of the public and the good of the individual, in fact, can be reconciled and mutually reinforcing. Ultimately, even community-level action must be articulated through individuals and thus requires interpersonal skills, a hallmark of nursing practice with individuals and families, as well as public advocacy skills. Boards and coalitions are made up of *individuals* who write letters, engage in public dialogue, get elected to office, change policy, and create communities where all citizens are enfranchised and have a voice. Interpersonal communication is a transferable skill that can be used to engage strategically selected citizens. While there may be a lag and some temporary discord between the health of individuals and the health of communities, ultimately, healthier communities result in healthier people. This book intentionally de-emphasizes the care of individuals and families, not because it is not important, but rather to introduce students to a kind of nursing practice, focused on health rather than disease, on communities rather than individuals, and on strengths as well as failings. By suspending the usual orientation to personal health services, we empower nursing students with new concepts and strategies that will help them build sustainable communities and thus promote the health of the people who live in them.

This text truly is just an introduction to community and public health nursing. There is so much more to learn—political science, policy formulation, biostatistics, epidemiology, anthropology, sociology, environmental science, world health applications, occupational health, school health, communicable diseases, participatory research, and so on—all of which we encourage students to acquire during graduate studies. The rudimentary concepts and strategies of this text are offered to raise the consciousness of all nurses to become informed citizens, conversant with the issues that confront our communities, our country, and our planet, and engage them in the realignment of the current structures that are creating unhealthy behavior and health disparities.

We assume most men and women choose to become nurses because they want to help people live well. Our hope is that they will see the unlimited possibilities of nursing to change the world.

REFERENCES

Butterfield, P.G. (1990). Thinking upstream: Nurturing a conceptual understanding of the societal context of health behavior. *Advances in Nursing Science, 12*(2), 1-8.

Dreher, M. (1982). The conflict of conservatism in public health nursing education. *Nursing Outlook, 30*(9), 504-509.

Drevdahl, D. (1995). Coming to voice: The power of emancipatory community interventions. *Advances in Nursing Science, 18*(2), 13-24.

Freeman, R. (1963). *Public health nursing practice* (3rd ed.). Philadelphia: Saunders.

Institute of Medicine. (1999). *To err is human: Building a safer health system.* Washington, DC: National Academies Press.

Institute of Medicine. (2001). *Crossing the quality chasm: A new health system for the 21st century.* Washington, DC: National Academies Press.

Institute of Medicine. (2003a). *Health professions education: A bridge to quality.* Washington, DC: National Academies Press.

Institute of Medicine. (2003b). *Keeping patients safe: Transforming the work environment of nurses.* Washington, DC: National Academies Press.

Williams, C. (1977). Community health nursing—What is it? *Nursing Outlook, 25,* 250-254.

INDEX

NUMBERS

9226 Kercheval Street, 10

A

accidents, community health assessment, 174–175

activity plans, creating a culture-based health plan, 220

advisory boards, 238

advocacy
culture-based leadership, 225–249
case statements, 246–248
complexity of clients, 229–233
constituencies and coalitions, 233–238
healthy community agenda, 238–246
implementation strategies, 226–229
culture-based planning, 199–222
community participation, 210–213
creating a plan, 213–222
population-based planning versus, 205–207
resource-based planning versus, 202–205
trends, 201–202
value of, 200–201

age of residents, community cultural assessment, 82–84

age-adjusted rates. See standardized rates

agencies (healthy planning), community health prevention infrastructure, 187

Agency for Toxic Substances and Disease Registry (ATSDR), 167

air pollution, community health assessment, 156–158

alternative health systems, community health prevention infrastructure, 190–191

American Nurses Association. See ANA

American Public Health Association. See APHA

ANA (American Nurses Association)
delineation of public and community health nursing, 39–43
national consensus conference, 40
Scope and Standards of Public Health Nursing Practice, 42

analysis
community health practice, 30–31
data analysis, community cultural assessment, 60–61
health analysis, community health assessment, 124

Annual Implementation Plan, 204

anthropological approach to medicine, 11–13

APHA (American Public Health Association)
delineation of public and community health nursing, 39–43
national consensus conference, 40

Arensberg, Conrad, 52

assessment
community cultural assessment, 51–118
analysis of data, 60–61
community as a place in time, 61
data collection, 54–58
population data, 80–90
process, 54
recording data, 58–60
social systems, 91–112
sources of data, 55–58
spatial dimensions, 62–72
temporal dimensions, 73–80
community health assessment, 119–191
analysis of health, 124
biostatistical measures, 125–130
defining healthy community, 120
environment, 154–161, 169–179
epidemiological studies, 130–133
indicators of health status, 146–154

measurements of health, 120–123
    population health, 124–125
    vulnerable groups, 134–145
    waste management, 161–168
  community health practice, 30–31
assurance activities, 41
ATSDR (Agency for Toxic Substances and
    Disease Registry), 167
attack rate (incidence), 129

B

behavioral health, community health assessment,
    138–139
beliefs about public health, 188–190
biological composition, community cultural
    assessment, 82–84
biostatistical measures, community health assess-
    ment, 125–130
    calculating rates, 125–130
    crude rates, 126
    morbidity rates, 128–130
    mortality rates, 127–128
    standardized rates, 126
boards of health (health departments), 185
boundaries of community, community cultural
    assessment, 62–63
breeding groups, 85

C

calculating rates, biostatistical measures,
    125–130
caring (concept of), application in public health, 9
case statements, culture-based leadership,
    246–248
case-control studies, community health assess-
    ment, 130–131
caseloads, 39
catchment areas, 26
CDC (Centers for Disease Control and
    Prevention), 152
census (United States), as population health sta-
    tus indicator, 151–152

Centers for Disease Control and Prevention
    (CDC), 152
chambers of commerce, community cultural
    assessment, 107
chemical waste, 166–167
chronic disability, 137
chronic diseases, 136–137
class, community cultural assessment, 67
clients, community health nursing, 25–28
climate factors, community cultural assessment,
    65
coalitions, culture-based leadership, 233–238
cohort studies, community health assessment,
    132–133
collection of data, community cultural assess-
    ment, 54–58
common good, community nursing values and
    conflicts, 35–37
communication patterns, cultural assessment,
    69–71
communities
    advisory boards, 238
    as community health nursing clients, 27–28
    culture, 24–25
    defined, 22–25
    environment, 24
    populations, 23–24
community cultural assessment, 51–118
    analysis of data, 60–61
    community as a place in time, 61
    data collection, 54–58
    population data, 80–90
        age of residents, 82–84
        biological composition, 82–84
        community as a population, 80–81
        education level, 87–88
        household characteristics, 89–90
        income level, 87–88
        management of population data, 90
        occupation level, 87–88
        racial and ethnic groups, 84–87
        residential characteristics, 89–90
        sex of residents, 82–84
        temporary subpopulations, 82
    process, 54
    recording data, 58–60

social systems, 91–112
    domestic organization, 97–99
    economic institutions, 93–94
    educational institutions, 102–104
    government structure, 94–96
    horizontal stratification, 108–110
    institutions, 91–112
    law enforcement structure, 94–96
    management of social system data, 112
    political structure, 94–96
    recreational activities, 104–106
    religious institutions, 100–102
    vertical segmentation, 110–112
    voluntary organizations, 106–108
sources of data, 55–58
spatial dimensions, 62–72
    climate factors, 65
    communication patterns, 69–71
    geophysical factors, 65
    housing patterns, 68–69
    land use, 66–67
    management of spatial data, 72
    mental maps, 71–72
    regional position, 63–64
    size and boundaries, 62–63
    topographical factors, 65
    transportation patterns, 69–71
temporal dimensions, 73–80
    community history, 73–74
    cyclical crises, 78–79
    cyclical population movement, 74–75
    economic cycle, 75–76
    management of time-specific data, 79–80
    psychological cycles, 76–78
community health assessment, 119–191
    analysis of health, 124
    biostatistical measures, 125–130
        crude rates, 126
        morbidity rates, 128–130
        mortality rates, 127–128
        standardized rates, 126
    community health defined, 20–22, 120
    environment, 154–161, 169–179
        accidents, 174–175
        air pollution, 156–158
        community buildings, 176–178
        crime, 172–173

disasters, 170–171
        disease vectors, 169–170
        energy management, 178–179
        food contamination, 160–161
        housing construction, 175–176
        water pollution, 158–159
    epidemiological studies, 130–133
    indicators of health status, 146–154
    infrastructure for prevention and promotion,
        180–191
        alternative systems, 190–191
        financing, 187–190
        health departments, 184–185
        personal services, 186–187
        planning agencies, 187
    measurements of health, 120–123
    population health, 124–125
    vulnerable groups, 134–145
        behavioral health, 138–139
        chronic disability, 137
        chronic diseases, 136–137
        infectious diseases, 135–136
        maternal-child health, 139
        maternal-child health behavior, 140–141
        school-age child health, 142–143
        unhealthy behaviors, 145
        worker health, 143–144
    waste management, 161–168
        chemical waste, 166–167
        noise pollution, 168
        radioactive waste, 164–165
        sewage, 163
        solid waste, 161–162
community health nursing, defined, 20
community health planning, 199–222
    culture-based planning
        community participation, 210–213
        creating a plan, 213–222
        trends, 201–202
        value of, 200–201
    population-based planning, 205–207
    resource-based planning, 202–205
community health practice
    action and advocacy
        culture-based leadership, 225–249
        culture-based planning, 199–222

cultural foundation, 19–47
    assessment and analysis, 30–31
    building community capacity, 28–29
    clients in community health nursing, 25–28
    community defined, 22–25
    community nursing practice, 29
    coordination, 32–33
    defining community health nursing, 20
    defining healthy community, 20–22
    evaluation, 33
    evolution of nursing practice, 37–44
    future of nursing practice, 37–44
    nurse-client relationships, 33–35
    nursing values and conflicts, 35–37
    planning and intervention, 31–33
cultural framework, 3–17
    conservatism in nursing practice, 8–10
    cultural competency in nursing practice, 5–8
    scientific basis of community health nursing, 10–13
community participation, culture-based planning, 210–213
complexity of clients, culture-based leadership, 229–233
Comprehensive Health Planning Act of 1966, 210
Comprehensive Health Planning and Community Health Service Amendments, 202
concept of caring, application in public health, 9
concept of community, 23
confidentiality, community health nursing, 34
conflict model (implementation strategy), 227–229
conflicts, community health nursing, 35–37
consensus model (implementation strategy), 226
conservatism in nursing practice, 8–10
constituencies, culture-based leadership, 233–238
coordination, community health practice, 32–33
cost-effectiveness, culture-based planning, 220–221
crime, community health assessment, 172–173
Crossing the Quality Chasm, 253
crude rates, biostatistical measures of community health, 126

cultural assessment of the community, 51–118
    analysis of data, 60–61
    community as a place in time, 61
    data collection, 54–58
    population data, 80–90
        age of residents, 82–84
        biological composition, 82–84
        community as a population, 80–81
        education level, 87–88
        household characteristics, 89–90
        income level, 87–88
        management of population data, 90
        occupation level, 87–88
        racial and ethnic groups, 84–87
        residential characteristics, 89–90
        sex of residents, 82–84
        temporary subpopulations, 82
    process, 54
    recording data, 58–60
    social systems, 91–112
        domestic organization, 97–99
        economic institutions, 93–94
        educational institutions, 102–104
        government structure, 94–96
        horizontal stratification, 108–110
        institutions, 91–112
        law enforcement structure, 94–96
        management of social system data, 112
        political structure, 94–96
        recreational activities, 104–106
        religious institutions, 100–102
        vertical segmentation, 110–112
        voluntary organizations, 106–108
    sources of data, 55–58
    spatial dimensions, 62–72
        climate factors, 65
        communication patterns, 69–71
        geophysical factors, 65
        housing patterns, 68–69
        land use, 66–67
        management of spatial data, 72
        mental maps, 71–72
        regional position, 63–64
        size and boundaries, 62–63
        topographical factors, 65
        transportation patterns, 69–71

temporal dimensions, 73–80
  community history, 73–74
  cyclical crises, 78–79
  cyclical population movement, 74–75
  economic cycle, 75–76
  management of time-specific data, 79–80
  psychological cycles, 76–78
cultural capital, defined, 8
cultural competency, 3, 5–8
  building community capacity, 8
  standard, 5
cultural foundation, community health practice, 19–47
  assessment and analysis, 30–31
  building community capacity, 28–29
  clients in community health nursing, 25–28
  community defined, 22–25
  community nursing practice, 29
  coordination, 32–33
  defining community health nursing, 20
  defining healthy community, 20–22
  evaluation, 33
  evolution of nursing practice, 37–44
  future of nursing practice, 37–44
  nurse-client relationships, 33–35
  nursing values and conflicts, 35–37
  planning and intervention, 31–33
cultural framework, community health practice, 3–17
  conservatism in nursing practice, 8–10
  cultural competency in nursing practice, 5–8
  scientific basis of community health nursing, 10–13
culture
  communities, 24–25
  defined, 6, 11
culture-based leadership, 225–249
  case statements, 246–248
  complexity of clients, 229–233
  constituencies and coalitions, 233–238
  healthy community agenda, 238–246
  implementation strategies, 226–229
culture-based planning, 199–222
  community participation, 210–213
  creating a plan, 213–222
  population-based planning versus, 205–207

resource-based planning versus, 202–205
trends, 201–202
value of, 200–201

D

data, community cultural assessment, 54–61
  analysis, 60-61
  collection, 54–58
demes (breeding groups), 85
Department of Health and Human Services, national consensus conference, 40
Department of Homeland Security (FEMA), 171
direct observation, as source of data collection, 56
disasters, community health assessment, 170–171
disease vectors, community health assessment, 169–170
disease-oriented funding programs, shift toward specialization in public health nursing, 38
districts (public health), 39
diversity, complexity of community clients, 230–231
Division of Nursing (Department of Health and Human Services), national consensus conference, 40
documents (community), as source of data collection, 58
domestic organization, community cultural assessment, 97–99
dose response relationships, 133

E

ecological fallacy, 7
economic institutions, community cultural assessment, 93–94
education level, community cultural assessment, 87–88
educational institutions, community cultural assessment, 102–104
energy management, community health assessment, 178–179
environment, 24
  community health assessment, 154–161, 169–179

accidents, 174–175
air pollution, 156–158
community buildings, 176–178
crime, 172–173
disasters, 170–171
disease vectors, 169–170
energy management, 178–179
food contamination, 160–161
housing construction, 175–176
water pollution, 158–159
Environmental Protection Agency (EPA), 167
EPA (Environmental Protection Agency), 167
epidemiology
as fundamental science of public health, 10–11
studies
as population health status indicator, 154
community health assessment, 130–133
espiritismo centers, 190
"Essentials of Public Health Nursing Practice and Education" (national consensus conference), 40
ethnicity
community cultural assessment, 67, 84-87
defined, 11
ethnographers, 12-13, 52
evaluation
community health practice, 33
culture-based planning, 221–222
Healthy People 2010 areas, 123
evolution of nursing practice, 37–44

F

family, defined, 97
Federal Emergency Management Agency (FEMA), 171
FEMA (Federal Emergency Management Agency), 171
financing (healthcare), community health prevention infrastructure, 187–190
Five-Year Health Systems Plan, 204
focus areas, *Healthy People 2010,* 122–123
focus groups, as source of data collection, 57
food contamination, community health assessment, 160–161

friendly societies, community cultural assessment, 107
future of nursing practice, 37–44

G

geophysical factors, community cultural assessment, 65
goals
culture-based planning, 214–216
Healthy People 2010, 1, 14
public health, 22
government system, community cultural assessment, 94–96
groups, as anthropological unit of analysis, 12–13

H

health assessment of the community, 119–191
analysis of health, 124
biostatistical measures, 125–130
crude rates, 126
morbidity rates, 128–130
mortality rates, 127–128
standardized rates, 126
defining healthy community, 120
environment, 154–161, 169–179
accidents, 174–175
air pollution, 156–158
community buildings, 176–178
crime, 172–173
disasters, 170–171
disease vectors, 169–170
energy management, 178–179
food contamination, 160–161
housing construction, 175–176
water pollution, 158–159
indicators of health status, 146–154
measurements of health, 120–123
population health, 124–125
vulnerable groups, 134–145
behavioral health, 138–139
chronic disability, 137
chronic diseases, 136–137
infectious diseases, 135–136
maternal-child health, 139

maternal-child health behavior, 140–141
school-age child health, 142–143
unhealthy behaviors, 145
worker health, 143–144
waste management, 161–168
chemical waste, 166–167
noise pollution, 168
radioactive waste, 164–165
sewage, 163
solid waste, 161–162
health departments, community health prevention infrastructure, 184–185
Health for All, 43
Health Planning Act of 1974, 210
health statistics, Internet sources, 147–151
Health Systems Agencies (HSAs), 203–204
Health, Culture, and Community: Case Studies of Public Reactions to Health Programs, 4
health-related data, community health assessment, 151–154
healthcare financing, community health prevention infrastructure, 187–190
healthy communities
agenda, 53, 238–246
defined, 20–22, 120
Healthy People 2010, 1, 14, 20, 28, 31, 49, 51, 53, 76, 81, 83, 85, 87, 91, 99, 104, 121-123, 134, 141, 154, 159, 173, 183-184, 186-187, 197-198, 214-215, 218, 226, 230, 253
healthy planning agencies, community health prevention infrastructure, 187
Hill-Burton Act of 1946, 210
homogeneity of populations, 85
horizontal stratification, community cultural assessment, 108–110
households
characteristics, community cultural assessment, 89–90
defined, 97
housing
construction, community health assessment, 175–176
patterns, community cultural assessment, 68–69
HSAs (Health Systems Agencies), 203–204

I–J

implementation strategies, culture-based leadership, 226–229
incidence (morbidity rates), 129
income level, community cultural assessment, 87–88
indicators of health status
community health assessment, 146–154
Healthy People 2010, 121
infectious diseases, community health assessment, 135–136
institutions, community cultural assessment, 91–112
domestic organization, 97–99
economic institutions, 93–94
educational institutions, 102–104
government structure, 94–96
law enforcement structure, 94–96
political structure, 94–96
recreational activities, 104–106
religious institutions, 100–102
voluntary organizations, 106–108
integrative model (implementation strategy), 226
internal diversity, complexity of community clients, 230–231
international health resources, Internet sources, 147–150
Internet sources, health statistics, 147–151
interventions
community health practice, 31–33
culture-based leadership, 225–249
case statements, 246–248
complexity of clients, 229–233
constituencies and coalitions, 233–238
healthy community agenda, 238–246
implementation strategies, 226–229
culture-based planning, 199–222
community participation, 210–213
creating a plan, 213–222
population-based planning versus, 205–207
resource-based planning versus, 202–205
trends, 201–202
value of, 200–201
interviews of community residents, as source of data collection, 57

K

Kiwanis clubs, community cultural assessment, 107

L

land use, community cultural assessment, 66–67
law enforcement structure, community cultural assessment, 94–96
local sources, as population health status indicator, 153–154
longitudinal studies, 132–133

M

management, community cultural assessment
  population data, 90
  social system data, 112
  spatial data, 72
  temporal data, 79–80
market populations, 26
maternal-child health, community health assessment, 139
maternal-child health behavior, community health assessment, 140–141
measurable outcomes, culture-based planning, 218
measurements of health, community health assessment, 120–123
medical anthropology, 11–13
medical pluralism, 190
mental maps, community cultural assessment, 71–72
MMWR (Morbidity and Mortality Weekly Report), 152
monitoring health, *Healthy People 2010* areas, 123
Morbidity and Mortality Weekly Report (MMWR), 152
morbidity rates, community health assessment, 128–130
mortality rates, community health assessment, 127–128

N

national consensus conference, Division of Nursing (Department of Health and Human Services), 40
National Disaster Medical System (NDMS), 171
National Health and Nutritional Examination Survey (NHANES), 152
National Health Survey, 152
National Institute for Occupational Safety and Health (NIOSH), 180
NDMS (National Disaster Medical System), 171
newly reported cases (morbidity rates), 129
newspapers, as source of data collection, 58
NHANES (National Health and Nutritional Examination Survey), 152
NIOSH (National Institute for Occupational Safety and Health), 180
noise pollution, community health assessment, 168
nurse-client relationships, community health practice, 33–35
nursing practice
  clients, 25–28
  community interventions, 31
  confidentiality, 34
  conservatism, 8–10
  cultural competency, 5–8
  defining community health nursing, 20
  evolution of, 37–44
  future of, 37–44
  political conservatism, 9
  role-modeling, 34
  scientific basis of community health nursing, 10–13
  values and conflicts, 35–37

O

occupation, community cultural assessment, 67, 87–88, 107
Occupational Safety and Health Administration (OSHA), 178
odds ratio (OR), 130
operational plans, culture-based planning,

219–220
OR (odds ratio), 130
OSHA (Occupational Safety and Health Administration), 178

P

personal health services, community health prevention infrastructure, 186–187
planning (community health planning), 31-33, 199–222
  culture-based planning
    community participation, 210–213
    creating a plan, 213–222
    population-based versus, 205–207
    resource-based planning versus, 202–205
    trends, 201–202
    value of, 200–201
  polarization, meeting needs of individuals and public, 254
  political conservatism, 9
  political structure, community cultural assessment, 94–96
  population-based planning
    culture-based planning versus, 205–207
    terminology, 26
populations
  as community health nursing clients, 25–27
  community cultural assessment, 80–90
    age of residents, 82–84
    biological composition, 82–84
    community as a population, 80–81
    education level, 87–88
    household characteristics, 89–90
    income level, 87–88
    management of population data, 90
    occupation level, 87–88
    racial and ethnic groups, 84–87
    residential characteristics, 89–90
    seasonal changes, 74–75
    sex of residents, 82–84
    temporary subpopulations, 82
  community health assessment, 124–125
  defined, 23–24
power model (implementation strategy), 227–229
prevalence (morbidity rates), 129

prevention infrastructure, community health assessment, 180–184
  alternative systems, 190–191
  financing, 187–190
  health departments, 184–185
  personal services, 186–187
  planning agencies, 187
primary prevention, 180–181
priorities, culture-based planning, 216–218
process, community cultural assessment, 54
professional societies, community cultural assessment, 107
promotion infrastructure, community health assessment, 180–184
  alternative systems, 190–191
  financing, 187–190
  health departments, 184–185
  personal services, 186–187
  planning agencies, 187
prospective cohort studies, 132
public health
  districts, 39
  goals, 22
  institutions, community health prevention infrastructure, 182–184
Public Law 89-749, 202

Q

QCPHNO (Quad Council of Public Health Nursing Organizations), 42
Quad Council of Public Health Nursing Organizations (QCPHNO), 42

R

racial groups, community cultural assessment, 84–87
radioactive waste, community health assessment, 164–165
rate calculation, biostatistical measures, 125–130
Rathbone, William, 38
recording data, community cultural assessment, 58–60

recreational activities, community cultural assessment, 104–106

regional position, community cultural assessment, 63–64

relative risk (RR), 130

religious institutions, community cultural assessment, 100–102

residential characteristics, community cultural assessment, 89–90

resource-based planning, 202–205

role-modeling, community health nurses, 34

RR (relative risk), 130

S

school systems, community cultural assessment, 102–104

school-age child health, community health assessment, 142–143

scientific basis of community health nursing, 10–13

Scope and Standards of Public Health Nursing Practice (ANA), 42

seasonal population changes, community cultural assessment, 74–75

secondary prevention, 180–181

secondary targets, healthy community agenda, 239–240

sewage, community health assessment, 163

sex of residents, community cultural assessment, 82–84

size of community, community cultural assessment, 62–63

social systems, community cultural assessment, 91–112
   domestic organization, 97–99
   economic institutions, 93–94
   educational institutions, 102–104
   government structure, 94–96
   horizontal stratification, 108–110
   institutions, 91–112
   law enforcement structure, 94–96
   management of social system data, 112

   political structure, 94–96
   recreational activities, 104–106
   religious institutions, 100–102
   vertical segmentation, 110–112
   voluntary organizations, 106–108

solid waste, community health assessment, 161–162

sources of data, community cultural assessment, 55–58

spatial dimensions (community), cultural assessment, 62–72
   climate factors, 65
   communication patterns, 69–71
   geophysical factors, 65
   housing patterns, 68–69
   land use, 66–67
   management of spatial data, 72
   mental maps, 71–72
   regional position, 63–64
   size and boundaries, 62–63
   topographical factors, 65
   transportation patterns, 69–71

specialization in public health nursing, 38

standard, cultural competency, 5

standardized rates, biostatistical measures, 126

state health departments, as population health status indicator, 152–153

statistics of health, Internet sources, 147–151

status of community, community cultural assessment, 108–110

strategic plans, creating a culture-based health plan, 220

surveys, as population health status indicator, 154

T

telephone directories, as source of data collection, 58

temporal dimensions, cultural assessment, 73–80
   community history, 73–74
   cyclical crises, 78–79
   cyclical population movement, 74–75

economic cycle, 75–76
management of time-specific data, 79–80
psychological cycles, 76–78
temporary subpopulations, community cultural assessment, 82
tertiary prevention, 180–181
To Err is Human: Building a Safer Health System, 253
topographical factors, community cultural assessment, 65
town nurses, 204
trade associations, community cultural assessment, 107
transportation patterns, community cultural assessment, 69–71
trends, culture-based planning, 201–202

U

unhealthy behaviors, community health assessment, 145
United States census, as population health status indicator, 151–152
units of analysis, groups, 12–13

V

values
    community health nursing, 35–37
    culture-based planning, 200–201
vertical segmentation, community cultural assessment, 110–112
voluntary organizations, community cultural assessment, 106–108
vulnerable groups, community health assessment, 134–145
    behavioral health, 138–139
    chronic disability, 137
    chronic diseases, 136–137
    infectious diseases, 135–136
    maternal-child health, 139
    maternal-child health behavior, 140–141
    school-age child health, 142–143
    unhealthy behaviors, 145
    worker health, 143–144

W–X–Y–Z

waste management, community health assessment, 161–168
    chemical waste, 166–167
    noise pollution, 168
    radioactive waste, 164–165
    sewage, 163
    solid waste, 161–162
water pollution, community health assessment, 158–159
wealth of community, community cultural assessment, 108–110
Web resources, health statistics, 147–151
worker health, community health assessment, 143–144